FOGSI EEBR 2025

Ethical Evidence-Based Recommendations

Antenatal Fetal Surveillance

Disclaimer

This Ethical Evidence-Based Recommendation (EEBR) document is drafted following a consensus between esteemed FOGSI experts and stakeholders and are based on the scientific evidence available at the time of preparation.

EEBRs should be used for information and educational purposes. They do not replace the need for application of clinical judgment to each individual presentation, or variations based on individual patient and resource setting.

Furthermore, EEBRs do not constitute or imply the endorsement of any of the included technologies, therapies, or techniques by FOGSI.

FOGSI EEBR 2025
Ethical Evidence-Based Recommendations
Antenatal Fetal Surveillance

Editor-in-Chief

Sunita Tandulwadkar

MD (Obs and Gyne) FICS (Gyne-Endoscopy) FICOG
President, FOGSI (2025–2026)
Gynecological Endoscopist and ART & IVF Specialist
Head, Department of Obstetrics and Gynecology
Chief, IVF & Endoscopy Center, Ruby Hall Clinic, Pune
Founder and Medical Director
Solo Clinic IVF—A Center for Excellence in Infertility and Endoscopy, Pune
Founder and Medical Director
Solo Stem Cells—A Stem Cell Research and Application Center, Pune
Founder and Director, Alive Regenerative Wellness
Pune, Maharashtra, India

Editor and Convener

Pooja Lodha

DNB (Obs and Gyne)
Fellow, Fetal Medicine, FOGSI-FMF UK Certified
Lead Consultant
Department of Fetal Medicine
Ruby Hall Clinic and Bharati Vidyapeeth University and Hospital, Pune
Director
Kangaroo Cradle, Fetal Care Centre
Pune, Maharashtra, India

Experts

Chinmayee Ratha

MS (Obs and Gyne) FRCOG (UK) FICOG FIMSA Diploma in Fetal Medicine (FMF-UK)
Director and Lead Consultant
Department of Fetal Medicine
Resolution Fetal Medicine Centre
Hyderabad, Telangana, India

Seetha Pal

DGO MD FRCOG FICOG RCOG/RCR Diploma in Advanced Obst Ultrasound
Senior Consultant
Department of Obstetrics and Fetal Medicine
Apollo Multispeciality Hospitals
Kolkata, West Bengal, India

JAYPEE BROTHERS MEDICAL PUBLISHERS

The Health Sciences Publisher

New Delhi | London

Jaypee Brothers Medical Publishers (P) Ltd

Headquarters
Jaypee Brothers Medical Publishers (P) Ltd
EMCA House, 23/23-B
Ansari Road, Daryaganj
New Delhi 110 002, India
Landline: +91-11-23272143, +91-11-23272703
+91-11-23282021, +91-11-23245672
Email: jaypee@jaypeebrothers.com

Corporate Office
Jaypee Brothers Medical Publishers (P) Ltd
4838/24, Ansari Road, Daryaganj
New Delhi 110 002, India
Phone: +91-11-43574357
Fax: +91-11-43574314
Email: jaypee@jaypeebrothers.com

Overseas Office
JP Medical Ltd.
83, Victoria Street, London
SW1H 0HW (UK)
Phone: +44 20 3170 8910
Fax: +44 (0)20 3008 6180
Email: info@jpmedpub.com

Website: www.jaypeebrothers.com
Website: www.jaypeedigital.com

Inquiries for bulk sales may be solicited at: jaypee@jaypeebrothers.com

FOGSI EEBR 2025—Ethical Evidence-Based Recommendations: Antenatal Fetal Surveillance

First Edition: **2025**

ISBN: 978-93-6616-060-3

Printed in India

Contributors

Chinmayee Ratha
MS (Obs and Gyne) FRCOG (UK) FICOG FIMSA
Diploma in Fetal Medicine (FMF-UK)
Director and Lead Consultant
Department of Fetal Medicine
Resolution Fetal Medicine Centre
Hyderabad, Telangana, India

Chitra Andrew
MD DNB MRCOG Postdoctoral Fellowship
Fetal Medicine
Professor
Department of Obstetrics and Gynecology
Sri Ramachandra Institute of Higher Education and Research
Chennai, Tamil Nadu, India

Geeta Kolar MD
Director
Department of Obstetrics and Fetal Medicine
Fernandez Hospital
Hyderabad, Telangana, India

Jaideep Malhotra
MBBS MD FIAJAGO FICOG FICMCH FICS FMAS FICMU FRCPI FRCOG FICMP FICRM
Managing Director, ART Rainbow IVF Agra
Director, Global Rainbow Healthcare, Agra
Director, MHMH (P) Ltd, Agra
President-Elect, In SARG
Past President, FOGSI, ISAR, ASPIRE, IMS, AOGS, SAFOMS, ISPAT
South Asia Director, IAN Donald School
Editor-in-Chief, SAFOG and SAFOMS Journals
Past Vice Chairman, ICOG
Immediate Past Chair, FIGO Committee of Reproductive Endocrinology & Infertility
Past Member
FIGO Working Group on RDEH
Director, SMRITI Manyata CSE
Founder, Club 35 Plus & Rotary Club Agra Grace

Kusagradhi Ghosh
MBBS MD DNB FICOG FRCOG RCOG/RCR PG Dip in Advanced Fetal USG
Consultant
Department of Obstetrics and Gynecology
Institute of Fetal Medicine
Kolkata, West Bengal, India

Mandakini Pradhan
MD DNB DM (Medical Genetics)
Professor and Head
Department of Maternal and Reproductive Health
Sanjay Gandhi Post Graduate Institute of Medical Sciences
Lucknow, Uttar Pradesh, India

Manisha Madhai Beck
MS (Obs and Gyne) FICOG
Professor and Head
Department of Maternal and Reproductive Health
Christian Medical College and Hospital
Vellore, Tamil Nadu, India

Meera Agalawe MS (Obs and Gyne)
Consultant
Department of Obstetrics and Gynecology
Siddhivinayak Hospital
Bhandara, Maharashtra, India

Narendra Malhotra
MBBS MD FIAJAGO FICMU FICOG FICMCH FRCOG FICS FMAS FIAPM
Managing Director
Ujala Cygnus Rainbow Hospital, Agra
Professor, Sarajevo School of Science and Technology, Bosnia
Director, Ian Donald School of Ultrasound, India
Vice President, World Association of Prenatal Medicine
Vice President, SAFOG (2019–2021)
President, In SARG
Past President, ISPAT/ISAR/IFUMB/FOGSI
Member, FIGO guidelines committee
Founder Editor, SAFOG Journal

Neharika Malhotra
MD (Obs and Gyne) FICMCH FMAS DRM (Germany) ICOG FRM
Infertility Consultant
Rainbow IVF Hospital
Agra, Uttar Pradesh, India
Chairman, FOGSI Youth Talent Promotion Committee (2020–2022)

Pooja Lodha
DNB (Obs and Gyne)
Fellow, Fetal Medicine, FOGSI-FMF UK Certified
Lead Consultant
Department of Fetal Medicine
Ruby Hall Clinic and Bharati Vidyapeeth University and Hospital, Pune
Director
Kangaroo Cradle, Fetal Care Centre
Pune, Maharashtra, India

Pooja Vaziraani
MD (Obs and Gyne) DNB Postdoctoral Fellowship in Fetal Medicine
International Masters in Maternal-Fetal Medicine (Barcelona, Spain)
Expert in Imaging in Maternal - Fetal Medicine (Barcelona- Spain)
Postgraduate in Fetal Cardiology (Barcelona, Spain)
Senior Fetal Medicine Consultant
Department of High-risk Obstetrics/Perinatology
Dr LH Hiranandani Hospital, NH SRCC Children's Hospital, Nidan Advanced Fetal Medicine Centre
Mumbai, Maharashtra, India

Prathima Radhakrishnan
FRCOG (UK) Diploma in Fetal Medicine (FMF, UK) Diploma in Advanced Obstetric Ultrasound (RCOG-RCR, UK)
Director and Consultant
Department of Fetal Medicine
Bangalore Fetal Medicine Centre
Bengaluru, Karnataka, India

Rachna Gupta
MS (Obs and Gyne) Diploma Fetal Medicine (FMF-UK) International Fellowship in Fetal Neurosonography (Israel)
Director
Department of Fetal Medicine
Sunehri Devi Hospital
Sonipat, Haryana, India

Sandhya Singh
FNB (Maternal and Fetal Medicine) MS DNB (Obstetrics and Gynecology)
Assistant Professor
Department of Maternal and Fetal Medicine
KMC Digital Hospital
Maharajganj, Uttar Pradesh, India

Seetha Pal
DGO MD FRCOG FICOG RCOG/RCR Diploma in Advanced Obst Ultrasound
Senior Consultant
Department of Obstetrics and Fetal Medicine
Apollo Multispeciality Hospitals
Kolkata, West Bengal, India

Sunita Tandulwadkar
MD (Obs and Gyne) FICS (Gyne-Endoscopy) FICOG
President, FOGSI (2025–2026)
Gynecological Endoscopist and ART & IVF Specialist
Head, Department of Obstetrics and Gynecology
Chief, IVF & Endoscopy Center
Ruby Hall Clinic, Pune
Founder and Medical Director
Solo Clinic IVF—A Center for Excellence in Infertility and Endoscopy, Pune
Founder and Medical Director
Solo Stem Cells—A Stem Cell Research and Application Center, Pune
Founder and Director
Alive Regenerative Wellness
Pune, Maharashtra, India

Uma Ram DGO DNB FRCOG
Director and OBGYN Lead
Seethapathy Clinic and Hospital
Chennai, Tamil Nadu, India

Vandana Bansal
MBBS MD DGO DNB FICOG FRCOG (UK) FNB (High-Risk Pregnancy and Perinatology)
Additional Professor and Head of Ultrasound
Department of Obstetrics and Gynecology and Fetal Medicine
Nowrosjee Wadia Maternity Hospital and Seth GS Medical College
Mumbai, Maharashtra, India

Preface

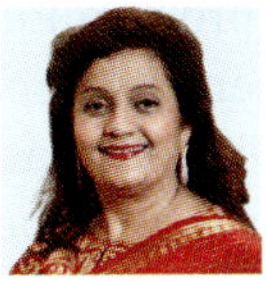

Editor-in-Chief
Sunita Tandulwadkar

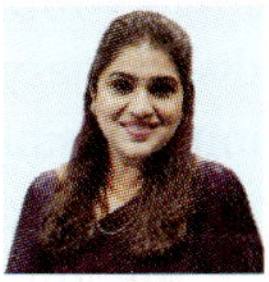

Editor and Convener
Pooja Lodha

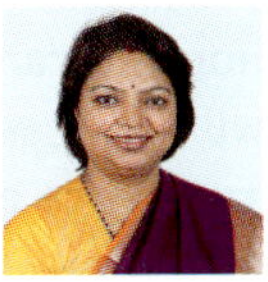

Expert
Chinmayee Ratha

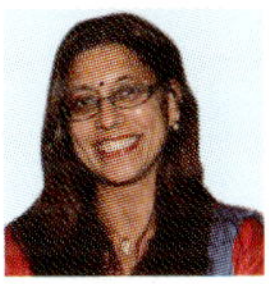

Expert
Seetha Pal

In our pursuit of advancing women's health in India, establishing our own ethical evidence-based recommendations is essential. As the President of the Federation of Obstetric and Gynaecological Societies of India (FOGSI) 2025, I am delighted to present this *Ethical Evidence-Based Recommendations on Antenatal Fetal Surveillance*, a comprehensive resource created through the collaborative efforts of dedicated experts across the country. While international organizations such as the International Federation of Gynecology and Obstetrics (FIGO), American Society for Reproductive Medicine (ASRM), and Royal College of Obstetricians and Gynaecologists (RCOG) have long established their recommendations, India has yet to create a unified, evidence-backed framework for fetal surveillance. This publication aims to bridge that gap, providing Indian practitioners with specialized, evidence-driven recommendations for optimizing antenatal fetal care in our healthcare landscape.

Fetal surveillance is a crucial component of antenatal care, particularly in pregnancies with elevated risks. These ethical evidence-based recommendations begin with amniotic fluid assessment, offering guidelines to evaluate and monitor one of the key indicators of fetal well-being. Subsequent sections address surveillance strategies for high-risk pregnancies, such as morbidly obese pregnant women and those with hyperglycemia, to mitigate risks and ensure safer outcomes. Additionally, dedicated recommendations for antenatal surveillance in dichorionic diamniotic (DCDA) twins provide clarity on managing twin pregnancies, where fetal monitoring needs are often more complex.

The publication further examines surveillance for immunologically positive pregnancies and pregnancies exposed to fetal teratogens, equipping practitioners with insights and protocols to protect fetal health in these challenging cases. A critical section addresses intrauterine fetal demise, offering guidelines to manage this sensitive condition with compassionate care and effective communication. Moreover, recommendations for fetal surveillance and antenatal counseling in pregnancies with surgically correctable fetal defects empower practitioners to provide timely interventions and informed support for expectant parents.

Guidance on fetal surveillance for pregnancies with "small babies" focuses on monitoring growth-restricted fetuses, aiming to improve outcomes through targeted care. The final section on USG and biochemical screening reviews key questions, recommendations, and evidence-based practices, giving practitioners a comprehensive approach to using diagnostic tools for early risk detection and assessment.

This publication represents FOGSI's commitment to equipping Indian gynecologists with the latest scientific advancements, framed within our cultural and clinical context. I am deeply grateful to the multidisciplinary team whose collaborative efforts have made these recommendations possible. We hope they become a trusted companion for practitioners, empowering them to deliver compassionate, evidence-based care throughout the antenatal journey.

Through this initiative, FOGSI reaffirms its dedication to advancing women's health and setting a new standard for ethical, informed care. We trust that these ethical evidence-based recommendations will serve as both a valuable guide and an inspiration for antenatal fetal surveillance across India.

Contents

CHAPTER 1

Amniotic Fluid Assessment

Pooja Vaziraani

INTRODUCTION

Amniotic fluid assessment is part of every obstetric ultrasound. Abnormal amniotic fluid volume (AFV) is a marker for a variety of pregnancy complications, including premature rupture, congenital anomalies, and placental dysfunction. Abnormal AFV leads to increased risk of complications such as umbilical cord compression, fetal deformation, fetal demise, and postpartum uterine atony (ISUOG, RCOG FGR guidelines, and BCnatal protocol). It also forms part of the biophysical profile and the "modified biophysical profile" in the 3rd trimester of pregnancy.

KEY QUESTIONS

1. Why and when does the amniotic fluid need to be assessed?
2. How do we assess and report the amniotic fluid volume at different stages of pregnancy?
3. How do we approach a case of oligohydramnios?
4. How do we approach a case with polyhydramnios?

Q1. Why and when does the amniotic fluid need to be assessed?

Draft recommendations:

- Amniotic fluid evaluation is an essential part of the assessment of fetal wellbeing and a normal amniotic fluid volume (AFV) is a sign of fetoplacental health. In combination with other modalities of fetal well-being assessment, ultrasound evaluation of AFV provides valuable information about a variety of fetal, placental, and maternal complications.
- Qualitative/subjective assessment of AFV can be done in any trimester, however semiquantitative methods, such as single deepest vertical pocket (SDP) can be done from 14 weeks onwards and amniotic fluid index (AFI) can be done from 24 weeks onwards.
- Amniotic fluid volume assessment by semiquantitative methods should be performed for all patients in the 3rd trimester and all cases of 2nd trimester which have an abnormal qualitative/subjective assessment or categorize into high-risk pregnancy.

Summary of evidence: According to the SAFE trial, ISUOG, qualitative/subjective assessment of AFV is usually performed in the mid-trimester, when the uterus is not too large to divide into four quadrants accurately, making it difficult to avoid measuring the same area twice. If the subjective evaluation suggests either less or increased liquor, then semiquantitative methods should be performed. The choice of method to assess the AFV objectively, especially in low-risk pregnancies is SDP.

Q2. How do we assess and report the amniotic fluid volume at different stages of pregnancy?

Draft recommendations:

- Amniotic fluid can be assessed by using one of two semiquantitative methods—(1) the single deepest pocket (SDP) and (2) the amniotic fluid index (AFI).
- If the AFV is low, the SDP is preferred as the criteria for oligohydramnios, and if the AFV is high, the AFI is preferred as a criterion for polyhydramnios. SDP is also preferred as a semi quantitative method in pregnancies between 14 and 20 weeks.
- *Thresholds for the SDP method:*
  - *Oligohydramnios:* Depth <2 cm
  - *Normal:* Depth ≥2 cm <8 cm
  - *Polyhydramnios:* Depth ≥8 cm
- *Thresholds for the AFI method:*
  - *Oligohydramnios:* AFI ≤5 cm
  - *Normal:* AFI >5 cm and <24 cm
  - *Polyhydramnios:* AFI ≥24–25 cm

Technical considerations needed while assessing the SDP or AFI:

- For SDP measure the maximum vertical column of fluid with a width of 1 cm and free of fetal parts and umbilical cord.
- For AFI divide the uterus into four quadrants using two perpendicular lines on the maternal abdomen. The longitudinal midline and the transverse midline between the pubic symphysis and fundus. Measure the maximum vertical column of fluid with a width of at least 1 cm, free from fetal parts and umbilical cord, in each quadrant. The final AFI is the sum of these measurements.
- Hold the ultrasound transducer perpendicular to the maternal position.
- Identify clear boundaries of the upper and lower edges of the pocket.
- Measure the largest unobstructed amniotic fluid pocket.
- Use color Doppler for areas where the umbilical cord is not visualized clearly.

Summary of evidence: The methods and technical aspects of amniotic fluid assessment are given in ISUOG mid-trimester scan guidelines 2018.

Evidence gap: The SAFE trial revealed that incorporating Amniotic Fluid Index (AFI) into routine obstetric assessments, particularly in low-risk populations, leads to, overdiagnosis of oligohydramnios, increased inductions, no significant improvement in maternal or fetal outcomes. Thus, AFI may not be useful for improving outcomes in low-risk pregnancies, and its use may lead to unnecessary interventions.

As per ISUOG, SAFE trial and the *Cochrane Database Syst Rev* 2008, both methods have a low sensitivity in diagnosing abnormal amniotic fluid volume as compared to dye-determination methods. Research studies suggest that the choice of measurement method should be tailored to the specific clinical concern, with DVP preferred for detecting oligohydramnios and AFI preferred for detecting polyhydramnios.

Q3. How do we approach a case of oligohydramnios?

Draft recommendations:

Maternal Evaluation:

- *Detailed maternal history and clinical evaluation:* Rule out drug intake and prelabor rupture of membranes.
- Measure blood pressure
- *Maternal serology:* Rule out infections

Fetal Evaluation

- Perform detailed ultrasound scan.
- Consider invasive procedures (amniocentesis) in certain cases.

Clinical management

- Follow appropriate protocols for PROM, IUGR, and management specific for fetal structural malformations and infections.
- Discontinue intake of drugs, especially prostaglandin synthesis inhibitors.
- Evaluate ductus arteriosus and tricuspid flow if necessary, in cases of drug-induced oligohydramnios and premature closure of membranes.
- Follow-up with weekly Doppler study from 28 weeks with expectant management till 37 weeks provided there is fetal wellbeing.
- There is currently no evidence to evaluate the use of transabdominal amnioinfusion in women with oligohydramnios secondary to rupture of fetal membranes before 26 weeks for improving perinatal outcome.

Summary of evidence: The management of oligohydramnios is cause-specific management (BCnatal protocol on singleton 2018, SAFE, Rabie et al. 2020).

Evidence gap: Further research is necessary to draw definitive conclusions on maternal hydration by oral or intravenous approach.

Q4. How do we approach a case with polyhydramnios?

Draft recommendations: The diagnosis of polyhydramnios should be defined as DVP ≥8 cm and AFI ≥25 cm is detected.

Three levels of severity are defined:
1. *AFI 25–29 cm:* Mild polyhydramnios
2. *AFI 30–34 cm:* Moderate polyhydramnios
3. *AFI ≥35 cm:* Severe polyhydramnios

Diagnostic workup for polyhydramnios depends on the etiological factors:
Rule out diabetes and isoimmunization:
- Assess anemia
- Rule out infectious causes
- Rule out malformative pathology
- Genetic assessment
- Label as idiopathic if the above test results are normal

Diagnostic amniotic fluid work-up should include:
- QF-PCR + CGH array + storage of DNA
- PCR for Parvo virus B19, CMV, Toxoplasmosis if maternal IgG positive or in the presence of fetal anemia of non-immune etiology.
- If tubulopathy (e.g., Bartter syndrome) is suspected then consider measuring the amniotic fluid levels of chlorine to rule out tubulopathy
- Consider a genetic study of myotonic dystrophy (e.g., Steinert disease) if suspected by reduced fetal movements or maternal phenotype.
- Additional amniotic fluid should be stored for possible further studies

Polyhydramnios is monitored according to its severity:
- Two weekly monitoring for mild cases
- Once a week monitoring for moderate to severe cases. In each visit the cervical length should also be assessed.
- If the moderate cases are stable with normal laboratory tests—the monitoring can be biweekly.
- Women with severe polyhydramnios should be delivered at a tertiary center due to the possibility that undiagnosed fetal anomalies may be present, e.g., upper GI malformations.

Summary of evidence: ACOG guideline and the SFMF consult series on polyhydramnios is categorized as mild, moderate, or severe based on amniotic fluid levels.

Even when apparently isolated polyhydramnios is associated with increased risk of perinatal complications. A recent meta-analysis pooling data from 2,392 patients with idiopathic polyhydramnios and 1,60,135 patients with normal amniotic fluid volume showed that the former was at higher risk of neonatal death (odds ratio (OR), 8.7), intrauterine fetal demise (OR, 7.6), NICU admission (OR, 1.9), macrosomia (OR, 2.9) and cesarean birth (OR, 2.3).

Evidence gap: ACOG and SFMF 2018 guidelines do not recommend antepartum fetal surveillance for isolated polyhydramnios. Despite common practice, there is no evidence that surveillance improves outcomes or reduces perinatal mortality in these cases.

BIBLIOGRAPHY

1. BCNATAL protocols on singleton polyhydramnios.
2. Gizzo S, Noventa M, Vitagliano A, et al. An Update on Maternal Hydration Strategies for Amniotic Fluid Improvement in Isolated Oligohydramnios and Normohydramnios: Evidence from a Systematic Review of Literature and Meta-Analysis. Plos One. 2015;10(12):e0144334.
3. Gu W, Zhao X, Wu Y, et al. Original Research: Amnioinfusion for the Management of Severe Oligohydramnios during the Second Trimester: A Retrospective Observational Study. Clin Exp Obstet Gynecol. 2023;50(7):145.
4. Kehl S, Schelkle A, Thomas A, et al. Single deepest vertical pocket or amniotic fluid index as evaluation test for predicting adverse pregnancy outcome (SAFE trial): a multicenter, open-label, randomized controlled trial. Ultrasound Obstet Gynecol. 2016;47(6):674-9.
5. Khalil A, Sotiriadis A, Chaoui R, et al. ISUOG Practice Guidelines: role of ultrasound in congenital infection. Ultrasound Obstet Gynecol. 2020.
6. Khalil A, Sotiriadis A, D'Antonio F, et al. Salomon, ISUOG Practice Guidelines: performance of third-trimester obstetric ultrasound scan. Ultrasound Obstet Gynecol. 2024.
7. Lees CC, Stampalija T, Baschat AA, et al. ISUOG Practice Guidelines: diagnosis and management of small-for-gestational-age fetus and fetal growth restriction. Ultrasound Obstet Gynecol. 2020.
8. Martínez J, Figueras F, Meler E, et al. BCnatal protocols on oligohydramnios in singleton gestation.
9. Pagan M, Magann EF, Rabie N, et al. Idiopathic polyhydramnios and pregnancy outcomes: systematic review and meta-analysis. Ultrasound Obstet Gynecol. 2022;61:302-9.
10. Prelabor Rupture of Membranes: ACOG Practice Bulletin, Number 217. Obstet Gynecol. 2018.
11. Rabie N, Magann E, Steelman S. Oligohydramnios in complicated and uncomplicated pregnancy: a systematic review and meta-analysis. Ultrasound Obstet Gynecol. 2017;49(4):442-9.
12. Rossi AC, Prefumo F. Perinatal outcomes of isolated oligohydramnios at term and post-term pregnancy: a systematic review of literature with meta-analysis. Eur J Obstet Gynecol Reprod Biol. 2013;169(2):149-54.
13. Salomon LJ, Alfirevic Z, Berghella V, et al. ISUOG Practice Guidelines (updated): performance of the routine mid-trimester fetal ultrasound scan. Ultrasound Obstet Gynecol. 2022.
14. Society for Maternal-Fetal Medicine (SMFM), Dashe JS, Pressman EK, et al. SMFM Consult Series #46: Evaluation and management of polyhydramnios. Am J Obstet Gynecol. 2018;219(4):B2-B8.

CHAPTER 2

Antenatal Surveillance for the Morbidly Obese Pregnant Woman

Geeta Kolar

INTRODUCTION

Obesity is recognized by the World Health Organization (WHO) as a disease in its own right. Moreover, obesity is an increasingly concerning public health issue across the world and its prevalence is rising amongst women of reproductive age. Obesity in pregnancy presents special challenges and limitations in prenatal care and increases the rate of pregnancy complications as well as complications later in life for both mother and child.

KEY QUESTIONS

1. How is obesity defined in pregnancy and classified?
2. Is obesity associated with increased maternal and foetal complications?
3. What is the Ideal gestational weight gain for obese women?
4. What is the specific nutritional advice for obese pregnant women?
5. When and how do we screen for diabetes in obese pregnant women?
6. How can we screen and prevent preeclampsia in morbidly obese women?
7. How do we screen and follow up for Fetal structural, chromosomal and growth abnormalities in obese pregnant women?
8. What is the risk of thromboembolism and recommendations to prevent thromboembolism?
9. What are the recommendations for management of labor, delivery and postpartum care in obese pregnant women?
10. What are the recommendations for pregnancy after bariatric surgery?

Q1. How is obesity defined in pregnancy and classified?

Draft recommendations: A pregnancy-specific definition of obesity has not been standardized, pregnant women are often considered obese/non-obese based on their prepregnancy BMI or BMI calculated at first antenatal visit (ideally by 10-week gestation).

Prevalence of obesity among women of reproductive age is increasing worldwide, with current estimates of 20–36%.

The most commonly used measurement for defining obesity is BMI, which refers to an individual's weight in kilograms divided by the square of her height in meters.

World Health Organization:

- *Overweight:* BMI between 25 and 30 kg/m^2
- *Obesity:* BMI ≥30 kg/m^2
- *Extreme/severe/morbid obesity:* BMI ≥40 kg/m^2
- *Superobese:* BMI of ≥50

Indian Asian classification of adult BMI:

- *Normal:* BMI kg/m^2 18–22.9
- *Overweight:* BMI kg/m^2 23–24.9
- *Obesity:* BMI >25

These differences in classification are reflected by the higher prevalence of gestational diabetes at a relatively low BMI for Asian populations than people of European descent and should be considered in clinical practice. The ideal management of this population remains a priority to improve both their own health and that of their future generations.

Summary of evidence: Obesity defined by Asian Indian guidelines (BMI ≥25 kg/m^2) is associated with adverse pregnancy outcomes at odds comparable to western studies with obesity taken as BMI ≥30 kg/m^2.

Evidence gap: *Pregnancy-specific definition* of obesity has not been standardized, pregnant women are often considered obese/non-obese based on their prepregnancy BMI or BMI calculated at first antenatal visit (ideally by 10-week gestation).

Variations in obesity—a significant proportion of the South Asian phenotype may have high body fat despite a normal body mass index (BMI), a phenotype called normal weight obesity.

Surrogate indicators of obesity like waist circumference, waist-hip ratio, neck circumference, waist-height ratio, and body fat estimation are not taken into account when we classify obesity based on BMI alone.

Q2. Is obesity associated with increased maternal and fetal complications?

Draft recommendations: Maternal obesity provides a major challenge to obstetric practice. Maternal obesity can result in negative outcomes for both women and fetuses. In utero fetal exposure to obesity appears to lead to metabolic syndrome in the offspring, which suggests the presence of a chain reaction that transmits the metabolic disease from one generation to the next.

The cause of adverse outcomes in obese women is uncertain. Causes of maternal obesity are complex and multifactorial. The increased risk may be due to obesity itself or the presence of comorbidities such as diabetes mellitus and hypertensive disorders of pregnancy.

Maternal risk	*Fetal risk*	*Intrapartum risk*	*Neonatal risk*	*Long-term risk*
• Hypertensive disorders • Gestational diabetes • Sleep dis-orders/ apnea • Depression	• Structural abnormalities • Twinning • Macrosomia • Growth restriction • Intrauterine death	• Increased risk of operative births • Anesthetic complications	• Asphyxia • Birth trauma • Sepsis • Hypoglycemia	• Reduced breast feeding • Neurodeve-lopmental outcomes • Obesity

Summary of evidence: The results of historical cohort study by Melchor in journal of perinatal medicine among singleton deliveries showed that prepregnant obese women have a higher risk of antenatal, intrapartum, postpartum and neonatal complications such as hypertensive disorders of pregnancy, maternal rectovaginal colonization with group B streptococci, induction of labor, cesarean section, repeat cesarean section in women with a history of cesarean birth, fetal macrosomia, meconium-stained amniotic fluid and infant admission to the NICU. In a recent study, Kim et al. found that the risk of any pregnancy complication was 18–47% higher among obese women.

Obese pregnant women are at increased risk of *maternal death* and complications during pregnancy and labor. In the United Kingdom, the latest Confidential Enquiry into Maternal and Child Health (CEMACH) reported that more than half of the deaths from direct or indirect causes during (late) pregnancy or labor were in overweight or obese women.

Evidence gap: Not all studies suggest that preconception weight loss, either through lifestyle or bariatric surgery improves fertility and pregnancy outcomes and support a causal link between adiposity and adverse pregnancy outcome.

Q3. What is the ideal gestational weight gain for obese women?

Draft recommendations: FIGO Committee guideline recommends that *all women should receive information on diet and lifestyle appropriate to their gestation including nutrient supplements, weight management, and regular physical activity.*

All women with obesity should be advised of the risks of pregnancy, childbirth, and long-term health.

World Health Organization body mass index classification and 2009 Institute of Medicine gestational weight gain recommendations.

	BMI	*Range of total weight gain (kg)*
Underweight	<18.5	12.7–18.1
Normal weight	18.5–24.9	11.3–15.9
Overweight	25–29.9	6.8–11.3
Obese (all classes)	>30	5–9

Summary of evidence: In 2009, the IOM (Institute of Medicine) revised the gestational weight guidelines on the basis of the increased incidence of obesity in women of reproductive age because obese women enter pregnancy with excess adipose tissue, the recommendation was to primarily meet the obligatory accrual of water and protein. Approximately 50–60% of obese pregnant women gain in excess of the IOM recommendations. Although some authors have suggested that less weight gain than the current IOM recommendations for obese women could improve some perinatal outcomes, inadequate gestational weight gain in obese women might have detrimental effects, including an increased risk of SGA infants, lower birthweight and fat mass, and potentially of greater consequence, a decrease in lean body mass, length, and head circumference. In general, inadequate weight gain and gestational weight loss should be avoided for obese women.

Evidence gap: There is a lack of consensus on optimal gestational weight gain. Until further evidence is available, a focus on a healthy diet may be more applicable than prescribed weight gain targets.

The updated IOM recommendations have met with controversial reactions from some physicians who believe that the weight gain targets are too high, especially for overweight and obese women.

Although both maternal obesity and excess gestational weight gain in a mother of normal pre-gestational BMI are associated with adverse pregnancy outcomes, obstetric management of obese mothers tends to focus on those who enter pregnancy being obese, whereas those who enter pregnancy at a healthy BMI but gain excess weight during gestation might not be as readily identified.

Q4. What is the specific nutritional advice for obese pregnant women?

Draft recommendations: Obese pregnant women should receive specialized dietary advice to counter the possibility of micronutrient deficiencies and allow for the added requirements of pregnancy. This includes a higher dose of folic acid (5 mg/day, from at least 1 month before conception and continuing during the first trimester) and vitamin D supplements.

Summary of evidence: International Federation of Gynecology and Obstetrics (FIGO) has highlighted the need to recognize maternal micronutrient deficiencies (e.g., iron, iodine, folate, vitamin B_{12}, calcium, and vitamin D) during all pregnancies, and to address these deficiencies through interventions including dietary diversity, consumption of fortified foods, and supplementation, as appropriate. Appropriate nutritional advice for obese pregnant mothers should also take into account cultural issues and diversity, and the fact that no single diet fits all is important to note. Because of the effect of obesity on the distribution and metabolism of folate, obese women can benefit from higher doses of folate supplements.

The RCOG green top Guideline on Care of women with Obesity in Pregnancy (2018) has highlighted the need of high dose folic acid and vitamin D supplementation.

Evidence gap: Various interventions, including diet, lifestyle, and drugs such as metformin, have been assessed with the aim to prevent or reduce obesity or excessive weight gain in pregnancy, and improve maternal and fetal outcomes.

The results of the Finnish Gestational Diabetes Prevention Study (RADIEL) of 269 obese women with a history of gestational diabetes, found that improvements in physical activity and dietary quality reduced gestational diabetes incidence, but again had no effect on maternal (e.g., preeclampsia, gestational hypertension) or neonatal (e.g., birthweight) outcomes. Interventions that are initiated before conception or during the first trimester might be more effective.

Q5. When and how do we screen for diabetes in the obese pregnant woman?

Draft recommendations:

All obese women should be screened for diabetes in pregnancy: Screening is recommended in the first trimester with fasting blood glucose and glycosylated HB (Hba1c) to rule out preexisting diabetes. Early diabetes screening at 16 weeks with 75 g is recommended for women with BMI >30 and repeat 75 g OGTT at 24 weeks if early OGTT is normal.

Criteria for diagnosing gestational diabetes (WHO):

- 75 g glucose any of the following
- Fasting glucose >5.1 mmol/L
- 1 h >10 mmol/L
- 2 h >8.5 mmol/L

Summary of evidence: Obesity is a major risk factor for gestational diabetes mellitus (GDM), associated with fetal macrosomia, as several studies and meta-analyses have demonstrated. A systematic review of the literature with meta-analysis by Torloni MR, calculated that for each 1 kg/m^2 increase in BMI the prevalence of gestational diabetes mellitus increased by 0.92%.

NICE Guideline on Diabetes in Pregnancy and SIGN guidelines recommend screening for all obese pregnant women for gestational diabetes.

Q6. What are the special considerations for screening and prevention of preeclampsia in obese women?

Draft recommendations:

- Appropriate size of cuff should be used for blood pressure measurement taken at booking visit and all subsequent visits. The cuff size used at the earliest point should be documented in medical records.
- First trimester assessment of uterine artery PI and biomarkers can be used for improving the sensitivity of screen for preeclampsia.
- Women with >1 risk factor for HDP and obesity may benefit from taking 150 mg aspirin from 12 weeks of pregnancy until birth.

Summary of evidence:

- FIGO recommends the use of an appropriately sized blood pressure cuff to measure blood pressure. Cuff size influences the accuracy of blood pressure assessment, especially in those with overweight and obesity. A cuff that is too small may overestimate blood pressure and lead to unnecessary medical intervention.
- FIGO also recommends that best practice for preeclampsia screening include additional risk assessments such as uterine artery pulsatility index, placental growth factor, and serum pregnancy-associated plasma protein A.
- Aspirin prophylaxis reduces the incidence of preeclampsia in high-risk women. Due to the increased risk of preeclampsia in obese patients, the German guidelines recommend administering aspirin starting in the first trimester in all patients with a BMI over 35 kg/m^2 as a way of improving pregnancy outcomes. Women with more than one moderate risk factor (BMI of 35 kg/m^2 or greater, first pregnancy, maternal age of >40 years, family history of preeclampsia and multiple pregnancy may benefit from taking 150 mg aspirin daily from 12 weeks of gestation till 36 weeks.

Evidence gap: The mechanisms linking obesity and preeclampsia are not fully understood, but it is thought that the metabolic alterations induced by obesity play a significant role. In higher-resource settings evidence for the applicability of these biomarkers in all populations and ethnic groups, and their additional role in improving early prediction of preterm preeclampsia is lacking. The relevance of these recommendations to LMICs is, therefore, uncertain and it is important that different countries modify the advice to be appropriate to the facilities and options available to them.

Q7. How do we screen and follow up for fetal structural, chromosomal, and growth abnormalities in obese pregnant women?

Draft recommendations: All pregnant women should be offered screening for fetal structural and chromosomal abnormalities. Obese pregnant women should be counselled that both ultrasound and blood tests for screening may be less effective in their case.

Fetal ultrasound assessments are recommended for:

- Nuchal scan between 11 and 13 weeks, 6 days
- Routine morphology scan at 18–20 weeks' gestation
- Fetal echocardiography with a review anatomy assessment at 22–24 weeks gestation
- Serial fetal growth scans after 28 weeks at 4 weekly intervals till birth (earlier if clinically indicated).

Consider use of transvaginal scan to help improve views as compared to transabdominal scans.

Screening for aneuploidies in obese women can be done by the combined FTS/Quadruple test with appropriate correction for BMI in the algorithms. If the cell free fetal DNA is used they may be counselled regarding a significant failure rate in obese patients due to lower fetal fractions. Patients with nonreportable cell-free DNA results should be offered diagnostic genetic testing, and clinicians should be aware of the increased risk of pregnancy complications in this group.

Summary of evidence: Maternal obesity can affect embryogenesis leading to congenital abnormalities, most particularly neural tube defects (NTD). Older epidemiological reviews have suggested an association of maternal obesity with various congenital malformations, such as spina bifida, heart defects, anal atresia, hypospadias, limb reduction defects, diaphragmatic hernia, and omphalocele. More recent meta-analyses have confirmed this associations for some conditions, especially for congenital heart disease and neural tube defects (NTDs), as well as for orofacial clefts and hydrocephalus, but not for the others.

RCOG GTG recommends screening by CFTS, Quad or NIPT with specific counseling in obese women. Patients with nonreportable cell-free DNA results are at increased risk for a number of adverse outcomes, including aneuploidy, preeclampsia, and preterm birth. They should be offered diagnostic genetic testing, and clinicians should be aware of the increased risk of pregnancy complications.

Symphysis-fundal height measurement is inaccurate for fetal growth assessment in women with a BMI >35 kg/m^2. These women should be referred for serial assessment of fetal size using ultrasound. Gaudet L, (2014) in maternal obesity and occurrence of fetal macrosomia—a systematic review and meta-analysis found an increase of 142% of birthweights over the 90th centile in obese women. The increase in neonates with a weight of over 4,500 g at birth was even greater (277%).

Evidence gap: At the moment, there are no consensus recommendations regarding screening options from scientific societies across the world on this issue.

In contrast to the clear clinical impact of macrosomia, the ability to accurately estimate fetal weight at the upper extremes is relatively low, with errors exceeding 10% of the birthweight. Significant refinements of EFW formulae are required to improve the accuracy of EFW predictions at the upper extremes of birth weight. It is important to inform the patient and her care team that the ultrasound evaluations may be limited, in particular on the basis of suboptimal visualization and inaccurate EFW at the upper extremes of fetal weight, to limit legal liability.

Q8. What is the risk of thromboembolism and recommendations to prevent thromboembolism?

Draft recommendations:

- Obstetricians should be aware that pregnant obese women have a preexisting risk factor for developing VTE - (aOR 4.4, 95% CI 1.6–11.9).
- VTE risk assessment should be done individually at all antenatal visits and documented appropriately-specific reassessments in this regard must be done intrapartum and postnatally.
- Obese pregnant women should be advised to be ambulatory and well hydrated throughout pregnancy.
- Pneumatic compression stockings on the lower extremities to be considered for all obese parturient prior to and during surgery as prophylaxis against deep vein thrombosis (DVT). The compression stockings should remain in place until the patient is fully ambulatory.
- DVT PROPHYLAXIS with low-molecular-weight heparin should be considered in women with a body mass index 40 kg/m^2.

Summary of evidence: RCOG GTG 126 (2018), 37a and b recommend screening and prophylaxis for VTE in Obese pregnant women.

Q9. What are the recommendations for management of labor, delivery, and postpartum care in obese pregnant women?

Draft recommendations:

Planning labor and delivery:

- Informed discussion with the obstetrician and anesthetist about a plan for labor and birth which should be documented in their antenatal notes.
- Elective induction of labor at term in obese women may reduce the chance of caesarean birth without increasing the risk of adverse outcomes.
- Women with a BMI 40 kg/m^2 or greater should have venous access established early in labor.
- Obese pregnant women should be made aware that they are at increased risk of stillbirth.
- Careful intrapartum fetal monitoring in labor should be provided.
- Obese women have a 2–3-fold increase in cesarean birth rate in both primigravida and multigravida women. This may be secondary to increased fetal size or maternal complications such as diabetes and hypertension.
- Active management of the third stage should be recommended to reduce the risk of postpartum hemorrhage (PPH).
- All maternity units should have a documented environmental risk assessment regarding the availability of facilities to care for pregnant women with a booking BMI 30 kg/m^2 or greater.

This risk assessment should address the following issues:

- Circulation space
- Accessibility, including doorway widths, and thresholds
- Safe working loads of equipment and floors
- Appropriate theatre gowns
- Equipment storage
- Transportation
- Staffing levels
- Availability of specific equipment, including large blood pressure cuffs, appropriately sized compression stockings and pneumatic compression devices, sit-on weighing scale, large chairs without arms, large wheelchairs, ultrasound scan couches, ward and delivery beds, mattresses, theater trolleys, operating theatre tables, and lifting and lateral transfer equipment.

Postpartum care:

- Women should receive appropriate specialist advice and support postnatally regarding the benefits, initiation, and maintenance of breastfeeding. Ongoing care, including postnatal contraception advice, should be provided to women with maternal obesity following pregnancy.
- An assessment of postpartum mental health should be done in obese women and appropriate referral pathways should be adopted in susceptible women.
- Maternal obesity should be considered when making the decision regarding the most appropriate form of postnatal contraception.
- Counselling regarding lifestyle modifications, Long term follow up for dyslipidemia, insulin resistance, hypertensive disorders is recommended maternal obesity can predispose their offspring to long-term health problems, potentially generating an intergenerational cycle of obesity and insulin resistance.

Evidence gap: There is insufficient evidence to recommend a specific lifestyle intervention to prevent depression and anxiety in obese pregnant women.

Q10. What are the recommendations for pregnancy after bariatric surgery?

Draft recommendations: A minimum waiting period of 12–18 months after bariatric surgery is recommended before attempting pregnancy to allow stabilization of body weight and to allow the correct identification and treatment of any possible nutritional deficiencies. Women with previous bariatric surgery should be referred to a dietician for advice with regard to their specialized nutritional needs.

This screening with an OGTT is *not* recommended for obese women who have had bariatric surgery especially malabsorptive bariatric surgery. In these women, the dumping syndrome makes the traditional glucose load unreliable as a screening test. For these women, in addition to fasting and HbA1c, consideration should be given to serial blood glucose measurements instead of the OGTT.

CONCLUSION

Maternal obesity in pregnancy is an increasingly common phenomenon and represents a significant threat to maternal and fetal/neonatal well-being. Few guidelines for management of this problem exist, and there is a lack of good evidence on which to base clinical practice.

In *early pregnancy,* setting guidelines for gestational weight gain through healthy eating and physical activity, and screening for fetal structural defects is warranted. In *mid-pregnancy,* screening for obstetric conditions, such as gestational diabetes and preeclampsia, needs to be initiated in all pregnancies. As gestation advances, *preparation for delivery* should include assessment for fetal overgrowth, timing of delivery, anesthesia consultation, and assurance that the delivery suite is appropriately staffed and equipped. Intrapartum decisions regarding the course of labor, caesarean delivery, and prophylactic antibiotics should be addressed. *Postpartum attention* in women who are obese should be directed to the increased risk of venous thromboembolism, difficulty with lactation, contraception, and depression.

BIBLIOGRAPHY

1. Athukorala C, Rumbold AR, Willson KJ, et al. Guidelines for the management of pregnant women with obesity: A systematic review. The risk of adverse pregnancy outcomes in women who are overweight or obese BMC Pregnancy and Childbirth. 2010;10:56.
2. Denison FC, Aedla NR, Keag O, et al. Care of Women with Obesity in Pregnancy. Green-top Guideline No. 72. BJOG. 2019;126(3):e62-e106.
3. Heslehurst N, Simpson H, Ells LJ, et al. The impact of maternal BMI status on pregnancy outcomes with immediate short-term obstetric resource implications: a meta-analysis. Obes Rev. 2008;9:635-83.
4. Kalra S, Kapoor N, Verma M, et al. Defining and Diagnosing Obesity in India: A Call for Advocacy and Action. J Obes. 2023;2023:4178121.
5. Maaeve K Hopkins MD. Obesity and no call results: optimal timing of cell free DNA testing and redraw. Am J Obstet Gynecol. 2021;225(4):417.
6. Ma RCW, Schmidt MI, Tam WH. Clinical management of pregnancy in the obese mother: before conception, during pregnancy, and postpartum. Lancet Diabetes Endocrinol. 2016;4(12):1037-49.
7. McAuliffe FM, Killeen SL, Jacob CM, et al. Management of prepregnancy, pregnancy and postpartum obesity from the FIGO pregnancy and non-communicable diseases committee (International Federation of gynecology

and obstetrics) Guideline 7. Int J Gynaecol Obstet. 2020;151 Suppl 1(Suppl 1): 16-36.
8. Melchor I, Burgos J, del Campo A. Effect of maternal obesity on pregnancy outcomes in women delivering singleton babies: a historical cohort study. J Perinat Med. 2019;47(6):625-30.
9. Misra A, Chowbey P, Makkar BM, et al. Consensus statement for diagnosis of obesity, abdominal obesity and the metabolic syndrome for Asian Indians and recommendations for physical activity, medical and surgical management. J Assoc Phys India. 2009;57:163-70.
10. Poston L, Harthoorn L, van der Beek E, et al. Obesity in Pregnancy: Implications for the Mother and Lifelong Health of the Child. A Consensus Statement. Pediatr Res. 2011;69:175-180.
11. Ramachenderan J, Bradford J, McLean M. Maternal obesity and pregnancy complications: a review. Aust N Z J Obstet Gynaecol. 2008;48(3):228-35.
12. Simon A, Pratt M, Hutton B, et al. Guidelines for the management of pregnant women with obesity: a systematic review. Obes Rev. 2020;21:e12972.
13. Torloni MR, Betran AP, Horta BL. Prepregnancy BMI and the risk of gestational diabetes: a systematic review of the literature with meta-analysis. Obes Rev. 2009;10:194-203.
14. Vitner D, Harris K, Maxwell C, et al. Obesity in Pregnancy: a comparison of four national guidelines. J Matern Fetal Neonatal Med. 2019;32(15):2580-90.

CHAPTER 3

Fetal Surveillance in Hyperglycemia in Pregnancy

Uma Ram

KEY QUESTIONS

1. What are the anticipated fetal problems that we should be aware of when managing pregnancy in a woman with hyperglycemia?
2. What are the most important aspects of ultrasound evaluation of the fetus in HIP?
3. How do we monitor fetal growth in hyperglycemia?
4. Can ultrasound assessment of fetal growth help improve glycemic control?
5. Is the risk of stillbirth more with HIP?
6. How can we optimize fetal surveillance in later pregnancy?

Q1. What are the anticipated fetal problems that we should be aware of when managing pregnancy in a woman with hyperglycemia?

Draft recommendations:

- Fetal complications from hyperglycemia can vary in severity and are directly linked to the level of hyperglycemia.
- The adverse outcomes from HIP include, miscarriage, fetal anomalies, stillbirth, fetal growth problems, difficult delivery, neonatal hypoglycemia, hyperbilirubinemia, and neonatal respiratory distress syndrome.
- The risks as well as the fact that they can be significantly reduced by good glycemic control need to be communicated to the woman and her family.

Summary of evidence: The risks for congenital malformations and some causes of perinatal mortality can be reduced to levels close to those of patients without diabetes with good glycemic control.

Q2. What are the most important aspects of ultrasound evaluation of the fetus in HIP?

Draft recommendations:

- Dating pregnancy is extremely important in women with hyperglycemia as they will have a planned birth. Additionally, these pregnancies are at risk of fetal growth problems.
- A late first trimester scan will be able to pick up a proportion of major fetal abnormalities and therefore needs to be done by a trained specialist.
- A detailed anatomy scan at 18–22 weeks along with a fetal echo is essential to identify fetal abnormalities.

Summary of evidence: Since women with hyperglycemia are likely to be delivered by 38–40 weeks, dating pregnancy is important and emphasized by NICE 2020. ISUOG guidelines on early pregnancy scanning (Salomon LJ et al.) give the recommendations on when the scan should be done. A detailed can in late first trimester is advised in these situations as they pick up a significant proportion of fetal abnormalities (Karim JN, et al.). FIGO, NICE, ACOG, and the Ministry of Health, India: Technical and Operational Guidelines as well as the Lancet series on GDM (Sweeting A et al.) suggest a detailed anatomy scan is advised between 18 and 22 weeks with a fetal echo as well (Bujitendijk et al.).

Q3. How do we monitor fetal growth in hyperglycemia?

Draft recommendations:

Timing of growth scans:

- In women with hyperglycemia, in high resource settings a scan every 4 weeks is offered to monitor growth.
- In limited resource settings periodic clinical assessment with accurate measurement of symphysis-fundal height and appropriate offer of growth scan is needed.
- In women on MNT with good control a scan at 28 and 26 weeks may be enough in contrast to women with poor control or those needing insulin/ OHA to achieve glycemic control.

Summary of evidence: Maternal hyperglycemia causes fetal hyperglycemia which in turn causes fetal hyperglycemia and fetal hyperinsulinemia. Once fetal hyperinsulinemia has developed, it increases the downward glucose gradient from the mother, to the fetus creating a fetal glucose steal. The result of increased delivery of maternal glucose to the fetus is fetal overgrowth.

Even though we are worried about fetal overgrowth and macrosomia, in reality fetal growth restriction is also possible and needs to be watched for. This could result from excessive calorie restriction in some women. It could also be a result of placental dysfunction. Therefore, where possible 4-weekly ultrasounds are recommended to monitor fetal growth.

Q4. Can ultrasound assessment of fetal growth help improve glycemic control?

Draft recommendations:

- Fetal growth patterns help identify abnormal growth patterns and are useful in the management of pregnancies with hyperglycemia.
- When the abdominal circumference/estimated fetal weight are >75th centile, it indicates a need to tighten glycemic control.
- When the fetal AC/EFW are on the lower centiles, it is important ensure adequate calorie intake as well as screen for placental dysfunction from other causes such as preeclampsia.

Summary of evidence: Kjos et al. proposed that the AC at 75th centile can be used to modify therapy in women with GDM. A metanalysis concluded that ultrasound-guided management improves birthweight distribution, but increases the need for insulin treatment.

Assessment of fetal growth starts later in the second and early third trimester, though there is evidence that fetal growth changes could predate a diagnosis of GDM when screening is only done at 24–28 weeks. Studies have also shown that in GDM fetuses which are appropriate for gestational age (AGA), there is increased subcutaneous fat deposition Longitudinal studies suggest that there is a biphasic pattern of growth in fetuses of women with obesity or GDM (Hivert MF et al.). Factors other than glucose levels, such as lipids, may influence accelerated fetal growth as evidenced by macrosomia seen in pregnancies with good glycemic control.

There is increasing understanding that there are ethnic differences in different aspects of GDM including fetal growth. Studies have shown that South Asian babies are smaller and exhibit a growth trajectory that is different from Caucasian fetuses (Venkatraman et al.).

Q5. Is the risk of stillbirth more with HIP?

Draft recommendations:

- Pregnancies with hyperglycemia are at increased risk of stillbirth. The risk of stillbirth is linked to the severity of hyperglycemia.
- The stillbirth risk is more in type 1 and type 2 diabetics when compared to gestational diabetes.
- Fetuses which are at the extreme of growth centiles (both LGA and SGA) are at an increased risk compared to fetuses that are normally growing.
- Risk of stillbirth can be increased due to other comorbidities such as obesity and preeclampsia.

Summary of evidence: Fetal compromise and stillbirth in GDM are linked to metabolic issues with hyperglycemia inducing the acidosis and cardiac dysfunction (Mathiesen et al.). Studies have reported a 4–6 times higher risk of stillbirth in the presence of diabetes than in the absence of it; 4% of all stillbirths are attributable to HIP (Starikov R et al.). Women with type 2 DM may be more affected due to the presence of comorbidities such as obesity, advanced maternal age, and hypertension.

The risk of stillbirth in women with GDM varies with the method of diagnosis, glycemic management and control, maternal comorbidities, and ethnicity. This could be the reason for conflicting data on the impact of management on stillbirth in GDM. The risk of stillbirth is impacted by gestational age and fetal size and increases over time to exceed the risk of expectant management at 39 weeks (Rosenstein MG et al.).

Q6. How can we optimize fetal surveillance in later pregnancy?

Summary of evidence: Most international guidelines mention initiation of surveillance at 38 weeks in women with GDM and this is incorporated in clinical practice. However, there is a paucity of evidence for the use of tests or a protocol for fetal surveillance such as CTG and biophysical profile for women with GDM.

The tools we have for fetal surveillance do not work effectively in GDM as tests of fetal surveillance identify placental dysfunction or pick up fetal response only after significant hypoxia sets in.

One observational study reported that cardiotocography could show changes suggestive of fetal hypoxia in births complicated by gestational diabetes, supporting the use of continuous cardiotocography during delivery (Tarvonen M).

Evidence gaps: There needs to be more studies to evaluate the optimal protocols for fetal surveillance in HIP. With increasing understanding of the role of other factors such as dyslipidemia and metabolic impact of hyperglycemia, alternate strategies to improve fetal surveillance and reduce stillbirth is needed.

There have been no large studies in the last decade to address issues around surveillance and timing of birth in women with hyperglycemia.

Hyperglycemia in pregnancy is a spectrum of disorders with varying risks that are based on the degree of hyperglycemia, its duration, and presence of comorbidities. We will need to evolve an individual approach keeping in mind the broad principles of care.

BIBLIOGRAPHY

1. Buijtendijk MF, Bet BB, Leeflang MM, et al. Diagnostic accuracy of ultrasound screening for fetal structural abnormalities during the first and second trimester of pregnancy in low-risk and unselected populations. Cochrane Database Syst Rev. 2024;5(5):CD014715.
2. Committee on Practice Bulletins-Obstetrics. ACOG Practice Bulletin No. 189: Nausea And Vomiting of Pregnancy. Obstet Gynecol. 2018;131(1):e15-e30.
3. Hivert MF, Backman H, Benhalima K, et al. Pathophysiology from preconception, during pregnancy, and beyond. Lancet. 2024;404(10448):158-74.
4. Hod M, Kapur A, Sacks DA, et al. The International Federation of Gynecology and Obstetrics (FIGO) Initiative on gestational diabetes mellitus: a pragmatic guide for diagnosis, management, and care. Int J Gynaecol Obstet. 2015;131 Suppl 3:S173-211.
5. Karim JN, Di Mascio D, Roberts N, et al. Detection of non-cardiac fetal abnormalities on ultrasound at 11-14 weeks: systematic review and meta-analysis. Ultrasound Obstet Gynecol. 2024;64(1):15-27.
6. Mathiesen ER, Ringholm L, Damm P. Stillbirth in diabetic pregnancies. Best Pract Res Clin Obstet Gynaecol. 2011;25(1):105-11.

7. Murphy HR. 2020 NICE guideline update: Good news for pregnant women with type 1 diabetes and past or current gestational diabetes. Diabetic Med. 2021;38(6):e14576.
8. Rosenstein MG, Cheng YW, Snowden JM, et al. The risk of stillbirth and infant death stratified by gestational age in women with gestational diabetes. Am J Obstet Gynecol. 2012. 206(4):309 e1-7.
9. Salomon LJ, Alfirevic Z, Bilardo CM, et al. ISUOG Practice Guidelines: performance of first-trimester fetal ultrasound scan. Ultrasound Obstet Gynecol. 2013;41:102-13.
10. Starikov R, Dudley D, Reddy UM. Stillbirth in the pregnancy complicated by diabetes. Curr Diab Rep. 2015;15(3):11.
11. Sweeting A, Hannah W, Backman H, et al. Epidemiology and management of gestational diabetes. Lancet. 2024;404(10448):175-92.
12. Tarvonen M, Hovi P, Sainio S, et al. Intrapartum cardiotocographic patterns and hypoxia-related perinatal outcomes in pregnancies complicated by gestational diabetes mellitus. Acta Diabetol. 2021;58:1563-73.
13. Venkataraman H, Ram U, Craik S, et al. Increased fetal adiposity prior to diagnosis of gestational diabetes in South Asians: more evidence for the 'thin-fat' baby. Diabetologia. 2017;60:399-405.

CHAPTER 4

Antenatal Surveillance in Dichorionic Diamniotic Twins

Kusagradhi Ghosh

KEY QUESTIONS

1. How is chorionicity determined in twin gestation?
2. How to screen for fetal aneuploidy in dichorionic twins?
3. How frequently should dichorionic twins be checked up in antenatal period, and how often should USG be done?
4. What is the role of fetal reduction and selective fetal termination in dichorionic twins?
5. How to manage single FGR (sFGR) in dichorionic diamniotic (DCDA) twins?
6. How should single fetal demise be managed in dichorionic twins?
7. When to deliver in dichorionic twins?
8. How to decide the mode of delivery in dichorionic twins?

Q1. How is chorionicity determined in twin gestation?

Draft recommendations

- *10 weeks or less:*
  - *Dichorionic:* Separate chorions around the individual gestation sacs.
  - *Monochorionic:* Single common chorion around both the gestation sacs.
- *11–14 weeks (most recommended gestation for determination of chorionicity):*
  - *Dichorionic:* Separate placenta, or Lambda-sign in adjacent placentae.
  - *Monochorionic:* T-sign at the membrane chorion interface.
- *>14 weeks:* (better avoided)
  - *Dichorionic:* Separate sex, or thick intertwin membranes in same-sex fetuses.
  - *Monochorionic:* Difficult to establish.
- If none is possible, assign as MCDA for antenatal management purposes
- *Nomenclature:* Membrane attachment is seen, fetus closest to the cervix is assigned as fetus A.
- *Monoamniotic:* No intertwin membrane. Single yolk sac suggestive of monoamniotic twins.

Summary of evidence: There was agreement among all international guidelines that chorionicity is best determined in the first trimester.

Pitfalls in determining chorionicity in advanced gestation include the disappearance of the twin peak sign (with regression of chorion frondosum) and, thinning of the intertwin membrane (Jing Lu). Intrauterine septum or synechia can be mistaken for an intertwin membrane (Jing Lu).

A review of 21 Clinical Practice Guidelines (CPG) concluded that the optimal gestational age for diagnosis of chorionicity is in early pregnancy, but their definition differed; most guidelines favoring 11–14 weeks (O Connor, Best Practice guideline). It is recommended to have a second opinion when there is confusion regarding chorionicity (O Connor).

Two yolk sacs in MC twins in early pregnancy should prompt to look for an intertwin membrane. Separate yolk sacs point to separate amniotic sacs but is not confirmatory (Ishii K).

Evidence gap: There is a difference in opinion regarding the timing of determination of chorionicity. Various nomenclatures are used in different national and international guidelines: "First trimester", "early pregnancy", "<16 weeks", and "11 weeks + 0 days to 13 weeks + 6 days". This needs to be standardized.

Q2. How to screen for fetal aneuploidy in dichorionic twins?

Draft recommendations:

- *Combined test:* Fetus A and fetus B may have different risks depending on the individual fetuses' CRL and NT measurements.
- Gestation age is assigned as per the date of ET (embryo transfer, +2) or BT (blastocyst transfer, +5). In natural conception with discordant CRL, with no obvious malformation, the gestation age is assigned as per the CRL of the bigger twin.
- Quadruple test is not validated in twins
- NIPT is better than other methods of screening for fetal aneuploidy in dichorionic diamniotic (DCDA) twins.
- NIPT has less sensitivity and specificity in DCDA twins than in singleton pregnancy.

Summary of evidence: The CRL of the larger twin should be taken for dating purposes (O Connor).

NIPT (cf-DNA) is superior to serum and ultrasound-based tests. cf-DNA analysis and ultrasound have synergistic roles in screening for fetal aneuploidy (Benn et al.).

In the case of fetal demise, anomaly or vanishing twin there is a significant risk of inaccurate test results following cf-DNA or serum-based aneuploidy screening (O Connor).

In the case of a vanishing twin, with a visible fetal pole on ultrasound, serum-based analysis is not recommended. Such pregnancies can be screened by NT and maternal age (O Connor).

Evidence gap: In the case of vanishing twins and early fetal demise, there is no consensus on when to do serum-based aneuploidy screening (both for biochemical screening and NIPT).

Q3. How frequently should dichorionic twins be checked up in antenatal period, and how often should USG be done?

Draft recommendations:

Uncomplicated DCDA twins:

- Four weekly till 28 weeks
- Two weekly till 34 weeks
- Weekly after 34 weeks till delivery
- Ultrasound monitoring of fetal growth every 4 weeks

Summary of evidence: ISUOG (Khalil) and most guidelines recommend four weekly USGs in DC twins to monitor fetal growth (Oliver); (O Connor).

Twin pregnancies necessitate closer antenatal surveillance. Evidence shows that following women with twins in a specialized twin clinic can improve obstetrical outcomes. The importance of the first antenatal visit in twin pregnancies is important for triaging and should preferably take place early in gestation (Hiersch).

Evidence gap: There is no agreement among international guidelines regarding the frequency of antenatal check-ups in dichorionic twins. The frequency of visits needs to be standardized, which necessitates further research (Hierch).

Q4. What is the role of fetal reduction and selective fetal termination in dichorionic twins?

Draft recommendations:

- *Selective fetal termination (SFT)—(where one fetus has an anomaly):*
  The indications for STF are:
  - One fetus with an anomaly that is lethal or likely to result in severe morbidity of that fetus/neonate, not affecting the other twin
  - One fetus with an anomaly that can jeopardize the other fetus (e.g., NTD, upper GI or respiratory tract obstruction resulting in polyhydramnios, which can cause preterm delivery).
- *Fetal reduction (FR)—(in uncomplicated dichorionic twins):*
  Indications for FR are:
  - *Maternal medical reasons:* Cardiorespiratory compromise of mother, e.g., high BP, COAD, or diabetes, advanced maternal age
  - *Couple's choice:* The couple already has one baby or cannot rear two babies due to lack of support at home or for financial reasons.

- *Which fetus to reduce in fetal reduction in dichorionic twins?*
  The reduction of the target fetus is dependent on various parameters. The target fetus is usually the one with the smaller CRL, the one away from the cervix, and the one easily approachable.
- *Which is the method of choice for FR in DC twins?*
  Intracardiac KCl is the method of choice. Other methods that have been tried are intracardiac lignocaine, digoxin, air embolism.
- Counseling is essential to explain the pros and cons and the procedure-related loss rate of up to 3–5%. An offer should be given to continue twin pregnancy even in cases with discordant anomaly.

Summary of evidence: Selective fetal termination refers to the reduction of an abnormal fetus (structural, chromosomal, or genetic) to improve the outcome of the normal fetus(es) in multiple pregnancies. Fetal reduction refers to the procedure of reducing one or more normal fetuses in multiple pregnancies, intending to improve perinatal outcomes or to ameliorate the socioeconomic challenges of delivering multiple pregnancies in the family (Sebghati and Khalil).

The findings of a systematic review (Sorrenti) show that, in dichorionic twin pregnancies, early ST (<18 weeks) is significantly associated with a lower risk of pregnancy loss and rates of PTB. An early anatomic evaluation of multiple pregnancies is therefore important.

Fetal reduction may be reserved as a remediation measure to improve the perinatal outcomes of dichorionic twins, only after thorough counseling (Jin et al.).

Evidence gap: There is a considerable evidence gap regarding whether fetal reduction in uncomplicated dichorionic twins improves perinatal outcomes or not, and hence, there is no consensus yet.

Q5. How to manage single FGR (sFGR) in DCDA twins?

Draft recommendations:

- Search should include an anatomy scan, screening for viral infections, an amniocentesis may be required to exclude chromosomal abnormalities (De Renzo, and ISUOG].
- Follow-up growth scans and Doppler studies of the FGR fetus are done to delay the delivery as much as possible (ISUOG).
- Umbilical artery, MCA, CPR, DV, AF volume to be done (AWM)
- *>34 weeks, and FGR is stage 2:* Deliver
- *28–34 weeks:* Close monitoring and, if required, in-utero transfer.
- *<28 weeks:* Thorough counseling and individualization is to be done regarding the various options:
  - *In-utero transfer to a higher center:* Delivery decision depends upon tertiary neonatal backup available there.

   - Continuation of pregnancy. Premature birth <28 weeks will put both babies at risk of extreme prematurity.
   - The FGR fetus, anyway, has higher neonatal mortality. Delivery <28 weeks will put the healthy fetus at risk also. The risks of long-term morbidity of the healthy fetus due to extreme prematurity (bronchopulmonary dysplasia, retinopathy of prematurity, developmental delay, neurobehavioral morbidity, and cerebral palsy) need to be explained.
   - Keeping the healthy fetus in mind, if the pregnancy is continued, the possibility of IUD of the FGR fetus is to be explained and documented.
- In case of elective premature delivery, steroids and magnesium sulfate are to be administered.
- Maternal medical condition, if any, gets priority over fetal salvageability. Counseling and documentation of the counselling, with proper consenting, are essential before terminating such pregnancies for maternal indications.
- It is better to seek a second opinion before delivering or continuing pregnancy in such scenarios of maternal/fetal conflicts.
- The mode of delivery in sFGR in twins is LSCS.

Summary of evidence: FIGO supports the use of a twin specific growth chart because "it may reduce unnecessary medical intervention", while most other guidelines supported using singleton growth charts.

On risk analysis, dichorionic pregnancies complicated by sFGR had a significantly higher risk of IUD [OR, 5.2 (95% CI, 3.2–8.6)] and composite morbidity or admission to the NICU, while there was no difference in the risk of PTB before 34 weeks or PE/gestational hypertension (D'antonio).

Evidence gap: There is no standardized staged-based management protocol in twins as there is for a single pregnancy.

Q6. How should single fetal demise be managed in dichorionic twins?

Draft recommendations:

- *Term fetus (37 weeks and above):* Deliver
- *34 weeks to <37 weeks:* If there is no maternal contraindication and the other fetus is normally grown with normal doppler studies, pregnancy is continued till 37 weeks.
- *28 weeks to <34 weeks:* The aim is to continue pregnancy as much as possible by monitoring maternal/fetal parameters:
   - *Maternal parameters:* BP, sugar, and clotting studies
   - *Fetal parameters:* Growth scans and doppler studies
- *<28 weeks:* Pregnancy continued as a singleton with monitoring of maternal and fetal parameters
- The risk of maternal DIC due to necrotic products of the dead fetus is low.

- The risk of prematurity remains high, particularly where the leading twin dies in utero.
- Delivery in cases of single fetal demise in late pregnancy is usually by LSCS.

Summary of evidence: The gestation at which single intrauterine fetal demise occurs, and the chorionicity of the multiple pregnancies, are the two most important factors when considering the risks to the surviving twin. Management should include fortnightly ultrasound scans for growth, umbilical artery Doppler studies, and liquor volume. With no other obstetric complications, dichorionic pregnancies can be delivered at term (Shek NW).

The timing of the death of the co-twin and the time of death have an impact on the outcome for the survivor. Compared to monochorionic twins the risk in dichorionic pregnancies is lower for neurological injury; however, the risk of prematurity remains high, particularly where the leading twin dies in utero (Eibhlín F Healy).

Evidence gap: There is no standardized guideline on how to manage such cases. The above recommendations have been drafted after reviewing several society guidelines and meta-analyses.

Q7. When to deliver in dichorionic twins?

Draft recommendations: Uncomplicated DCDA twin pregnancy may be continued till term (37 weeks). Delivery is better done between 37 + 0 and 38 + 0 weeks.

Premature delivery may need to be done depending on maternal and fetal complications, if any:

- *Maternal conditions:* Uncontrolled BP, sugar, respiratory distress, obstetric cholestasis.
- *Fetal conditions:* FGR, fetal anomaly, if any.

Summary of evidence: Out of 21 guidelines reviewed, 23.6% recommend between 37 and 38 weeks, one guideline recommends delivery at 36 weeks, 12% allow delivery beyond 38 + 0 weeks, 6% were vague and recommended delivery before 40 weeks, and 47% do not mention the timing of delivery (Oliver).

Evidence gap: A comparative review of National and International guidelines highlighted the differences in the management of uncomplicated and complicated twin pregnancies and the need for adopting an International consensus to improve perinatal outcomes (Tsakiridis).

Q8. How to decide the mode of delivery in dichorionic twins?

Draft recommendations: DC twins with first fetus in non-cephalic presentation; delivery is by LSCS.

In uncomplicated DC twins, vaginal delivery may be allowed if the presenting fetus is in cephalic presentation.

If the couple requests for normal delivery, they should be explained about the risks involved, especially to the second-born fetus after the delivery of the first. Counseling is important in deciding the mode of delivery. In complicated DCDA twins, the mode of delivery is by LSCS.

Summary of evidence: There is consensus regarding the vaginal delivery of uncomplicated DC twins when the first fetus is in cephalic presentation.

A total of 71% of guidelines recommend vaginal delivery if the second fetus is in a non-cephalic position, thereby allowing an external cephalic version and assisted breech delivery or internal podalic version and breech extraction, if required. 29% of guidelines were in favor of LSCS for DC twins when the second fetus is in non-cephalic presentation (Oliver).

Cesarean section delivery was recommended in DC twins in the case of a large head circumference or in the case of major obstetric risk factors (not defined) (O Connor).

Dichorionic-diamniotic twins should be delivered at 37 0/7 to 38 0/7. Breech extraction done by a competent professional may be allowed in non-cephalic second twin. Cesarean delivery is likely beneficial for twin pregnancies with the first twin in non-cephalic presentation. In all multiple pregnancies, delivery should be performed by an experienced practitioner (Aviram et al).

Evidence gap: There is no agreement among international guidelines regarding vaginal delivery in uncomplicated DCDA twins when the second fetus is in non-cephalic presentation (Oliver).

Whether to wait for the spontaneous onset of labor or to go for labor induction at term: There is no clear evidence or guideline on this issue (Oliver); (O Connor).

Future research: There is a paucity of robust literature on DCDA twins:

- There are more guidelines and protocols for managing MC twins compared to DC twins. This needs to be addressed.
- Management of discordant fetal anomaly or single fetal demise needs greater consideration within DC twins.
- Use of USG monitoring of cervical length in twins
- Vaginal delivery in DC twins
- Induction of labor, timing, and preferred methods of induction
- Mode of intrapartum fetal monitoring
- Cord clamping in DCDA twins

Despite advancements in USG monitoring of twin fetuses, lack of defined timings of delivery, and clear management strategies for the delivery of twins may lead to variable outcomes for women and their fetuses. This is not desirable, and more research needs to be done to address these issues.

BIBLIOGRAPHY

1. Aviram A, Barrett JFR, Melamed N, et al. Mode of delivery in multiple pregnancies. Am J Obstet Gynecol MFM. 2022;4(2S):100470.
2. Benn P, Rebarber A. Non-invasive prenatal testing in the management of twin pregnancies. Prenat Diagn. 2021;41(10):1233-40.
3. D'antonio F, Prasad S, Masciullo L, et al. Selective fetal growth restriction in dichorionic diamniotic twin pregnancy: systematic review and meta-analysis of pregnancy and perinatal outcomes. Ultrasound Obstet Gynecol. 2024;63(2):164-72.
4. Healy EF, Khalil A. Single intrauterine death in twin pregnancy: Evidenced-based counselling and management. Best Pract Res Clin Obstet Gynaecol. 2022:84:205-17.
5. Hiersch L, Attali E, Melamed N. Special considerations regarding antenatal care and pregnancy complications in dichorionic twin pregnancies. Am J Obstet Gynecol MFM. 2022;4(2S):100500.
6. Ishii K. Prenatal diagnosis and management of monoamniotic twins: Review. Curr Opin Obstet Gynecol. 2015;27(2):159-64.
7. Jin B, Huang Q, Ji M, et al. Perinatal outcomes in dichorionic diamniotic twins with multifetal pregnancy reduction versus expectant management: a systematic review and meta-analysis. Medicine (Baltimore). 2020;99(25):e20730.
8. Khalil A, Rodgers M, Baschat A, et al. ISUOG Practice Guidelines: role of ultrasound in twin pregnancy. Ultrasound Obstet Gynecol. 2016;47(2):247-63.
9. Lu J, Ting YH , Leung TY. Determining chorionicity and amnionicity in twin pregnancies: Pitfalls. Best Pract Res Clin Obstet Gynaecol. 2022:84:2-16.
10. Oliver E, Navaratnam K, Gent J, et al. Comparison of international guidelines on the management of twin pregnancy. Eur J Obstet Gynecol Reprod Biol. 2023; 285:97-104.
11. O'Connor C, O'Connor E, Leitao S, et al. Clinical practice guidelines for the antenatal management of dichorionic diamniotic twin pregnancies: a systematic review. BMC Pregnancy Childbirth. 2023;23(1):347.
12. Sebghati M, Khalil A. Reduction of multiple pregnancy: Counselling and techniques. Review. Best Pract Res Clin Obstet Gynaecol. 2021;70:112-22.
13. Shek NW, Hillman SC, Kilby MD. Single-twin demise: pregnancy outcome. Best Pract Res Clin Obstet Gynaecol. 2014;28(2):249-63.
14. Sorrenti S, Di Mascio D, Khalil A, et al. Pregnancy and perinatal outcomes of early vs late selective termination in dichorionic twin pregnancy: systematic review and meta-analysis. Ultrasound Obstet Gynecol. 2023;61(5):552-8.
15. Tsakiridis I, Giouleka S, Mamopoulos A, et al. Management of Twin Pregnancies: A Comparative Review of National and International Guidelines. Obstet Gynecol Surv. 2020;75(7):419-30.

5

CHAPTER

Antenatal Surveillance in Monochorionic Gestation

Chinmayee Ratha

INTRODUCTION

Monochorionic twins present a different challenge in antenatal surveillance as compared to dichorionic twins since there is a common placenta between the twin fetuses. This sharing of placenta becomes a unique reason for some specific complications in pregnancy and hence antenatal surveillance in monochorionic twins has to be customized to enable the clinician to suspect and detect these complications well in time to ensure reasonable management of the same.

KEY QUESTIONS

1. How often should ultrasounds be performed in multiple pregnancy?
2. What are the specific ultrasound markers to monitor?
3. How should growth discordance be assessed and managed?
4. Differential diagnosis algorithm for MC twins with suspected TTTS and/or sFGR.
5. What are the common available treatment options for MC complications?
6. Which are the common post treatment complications in MC (like TAPS)?
7. What are the best practices for coordinating care among the health care team?

Q1. How often should ultrasound be performed in multiple pregnancy?

- Uncomplicated dichorionic twin pregnancy should have a first-trimester scan, a detailed second-trimester scan, and scans every 4 weeks thereafter.
- Complicated dichorionic twins should be scanned more frequently, depending on the condition and its severity.
- Uncomplicated monochorionic twins should have a first-trimester scan and be scanned every 2 weeks after 16 weeks in order to detect TTTS and TAPS in a timely manner.
- Complicated monochorionic twins should be scanned more frequently, depending on the condition and its severity.
- *Uncomplicated, dichorionic pregnancy:* Visits every 4 weeks after first-trimester ultrasound until 32 weeks, then every 2 weeks until 36 weeks, and then weekly.
- *Uncomplicated monochorionic pregnancy:* Visits every 2 weeks after first-trimester ultrasound until 34 weeks and then weekly.

- *Uncomplicated triplet pregnancy:* Visits every 4 weeks after first-trimester ultrasound until week 24, then visits every 2 weeks until week 32, and then weekly. In triple pregnancies and monochorionic component, checkups will be fortnightly from the beginning until 32 weeks and then weekly.
- In triplet pregnancies with monochorionic component, ultrasound recommendations apply as in monochorionic twin pregnancy.

Q2. What are the specific ultrasound markers to monitor?

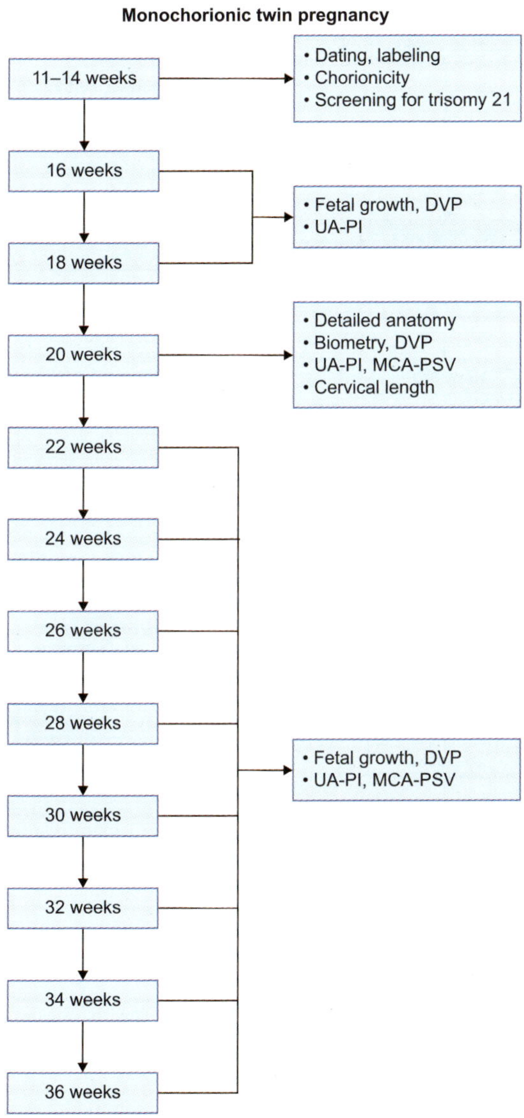

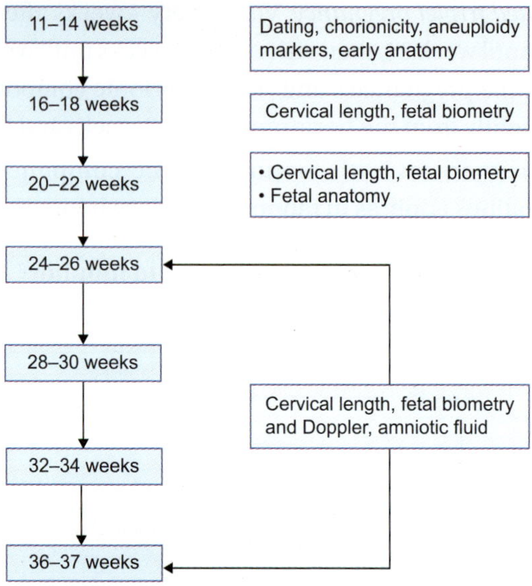
11–14 weeks
Dating, chorionicity, aneuploidy markers, early anatomy
16–18 weeks
Cervical length, fetal biometry
20–22 weeks
• Cervical length, fetal biometry
• Fetal anatomy
24–26 weeks
28–30 weeks
Cervical length, fetal biometry and Doppler, amniotic fluid
32–34 weeks
36–37 weeks

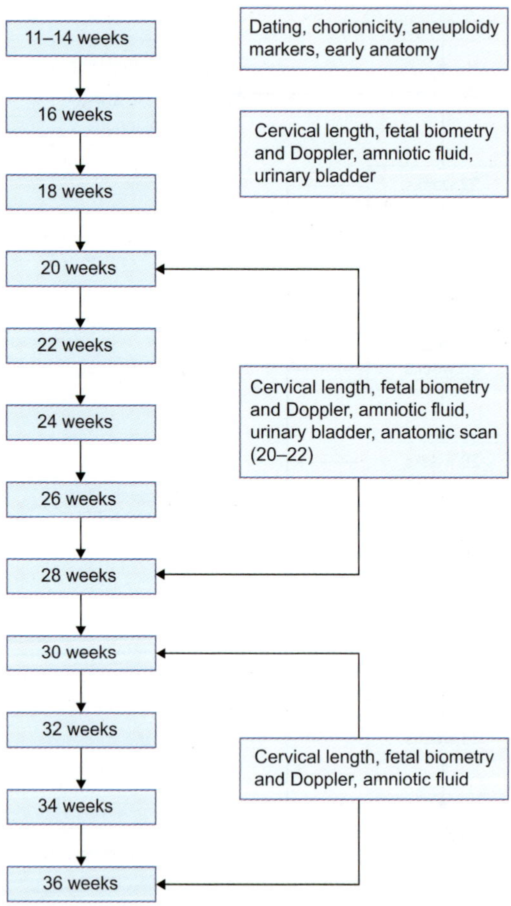
11–14 weeks
Dating, chorionicity, aneuploidy markers, early anatomy
16 weeks
Cervical length, fetal biometry and Doppler, amniotic fluid, urinary bladder
18 weeks
20 weeks
22 weeks
Cervical length, fetal biometry and Doppler, amniotic fluid, urinary bladder, anatomic scan (20–22)
24 weeks
26 weeks
28 weeks
30 weeks
32 weeks
Cervical length, fetal biometry and Doppler, amniotic fluid
34 weeks
36 weeks

Ultrasound objectives

- *Fetal growth monitoring:* Due to the increased risk of fetal growth restriction (FGR), percentiles and intertwin weight discordance should be reported at each ultrasound scan.
- Customized growth charts for multiple pregnancy (differentiating dichorionic from monochorionic charts) should be used.
- *Rule out specific complications of monochorionic pregnancy:* Early diagnosis of TTTS by monitoring amniotic fluid, urinary bladders, fetal Doppler, and biometry from 14 to 16 weeks onward.
- Early diagnosis of TAPS by monitoring middle cerebral artery (MCA) and peak systolic velocity (PSV) from 20 weeks onward.
- In all monochorionic pregnancies, a fetal echocardiography will be requested from 13 to 14 weeks, and another at 20–22 weeks, due to the increased risk of heart defect.

Q3. How should growth discordance be assessed and managed?

- Discordant growth is considered when the estimated weight difference is >20–25% based on the estimated weight of the larger twin: (Larger weight – Smaller weight) × 100/Larger weight.
- A weight discordance ≥25% is an independent poor prognostic factor associated with increased perinatal mortality and morbidity, especially in monochorionic twins.
- Fetal growth is considered restricted when the estimated fetal weight is below the 10th percentile.

Selective fetal growth restriction in twin pregnancy	
International Consensus: Diagnostic features	
Dichorionic twins	*Monochorionic twins*
Solitary: EFW <3rd centile	*Solitary:* EFW <3rd centile
Contributory: At least 2/3	*Contributory:* At least 2/4
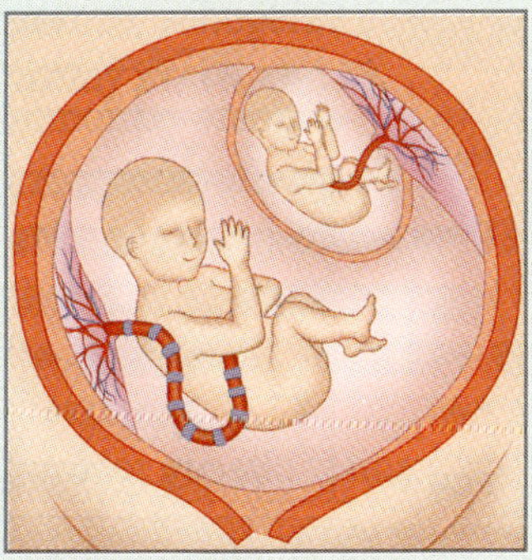	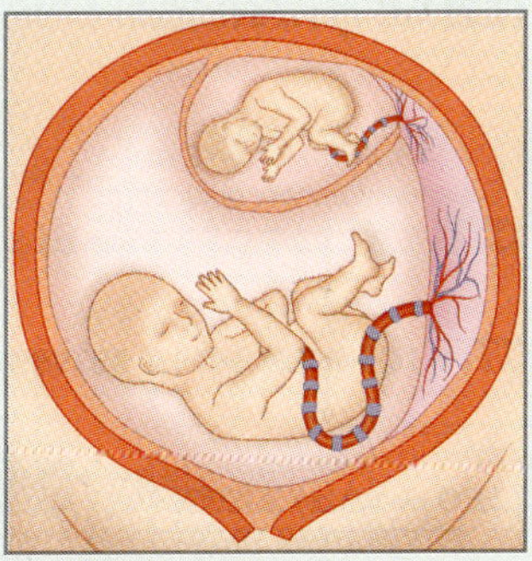
• EFW <10th centile • EFW discordance ≥25% • Umbilical PI >95th centile	• EFW <10th centile • EFW discordance ≥25% • Umbilical PI >95th centile • AC <10th centile

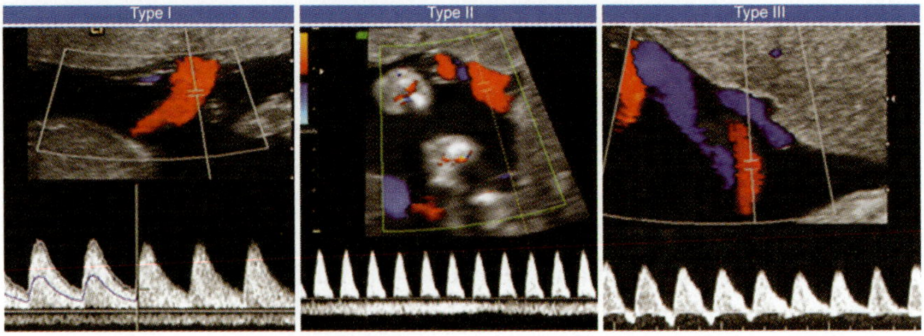

Fig. 1: Classification of selective fetal growth restriction in monochorionic twin pregnancy. In Type I, the umbilical artery Doppler waveform has positive end-diastolic flow, while in Type II, there is absent or reversed end-diastolic flow (AREDF). In Type III, there is a cyclical/intermittent pattern of AREDF.

Diagnosis of sFGR

- The diagnosis of sFGR in a MC pregnancy requires first ruling out TTTS.
- Amniotic fluid discordance is a common finding in sFGR, but the criteria for TTTS must not be met.
- It is possible to have TTTS and sFGR, but the case must be managed as TTTS.
- As a rule, the diagnosis of sFGR should be considered when one fetus has an estimated fetal weight <10 centile.
- This finding should lead to closer follow-up and Doppler examination of both fetuses and classification into types according to the UA Doppler of the smaller fetus.
- A more refined classification has been proposed according to combinations of criteria, but the clinical implications do not change in relation with the previous simplified criterion.

Q4. Differential diagnosis algorithm for MC twins with suspected TTTS and/or sFGR.

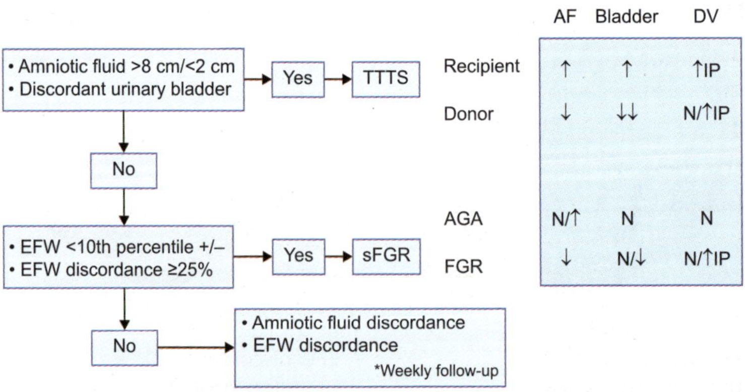

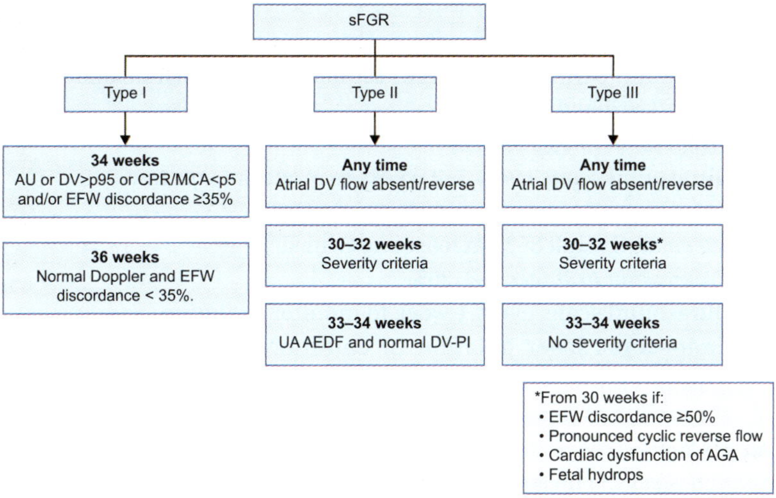

	sFGR	***TTTS***
EFW discordance	≥25% and EFW <10th percentile	Variable
AGA/recipient fetus:* • Amniotic fluid • Urinary bladder • Ductus venosus	 • Normal or slightly increased • Normal • Normal	 • >8 cm before 20 weeks • >10 cm after 20 weeks • Enlarged • Variable (elevated PI)
FGR/donor fetus: • Amniotic fluid • Urinary bladder	 • Normal or slightly reduced • Normal or slightly reduced	 • <2 cm • Very reduced/No visible

Q5. What are the common available management options for MC complications?

TTTS

- There is an imbalance in the net flow of blood across the placental vascular communications from one fetus, the donor, to the other, the recipient.
- *11–14 weeks:* Early TTTS is suspected if there is discordance in size of the amniotic fluid sacs, ≥20% discordance in fetal nuchal translucency (NT) thickness, or absent/reversed end diastolic flow (EDF) in the ductus venosus usually in the fetus with higher NT.
- *≥15 weeks:* Oligohydramnios (deepest vertical pool of ≤2 cm) in the sac of the oliguric or anuric donor fetus and polyhydramnios (≥6 cm at 15–17 weeks, ≥8 cm at 18–20 weeks and >10 cm at ≥20 weeks) in the sac of the polyuric recipient.

Management

- *Discordance in amniotic fluid* (but not sufficient to fulfill the oligohydramnios/polyhydramnios sequence) with normal fetal Doppler:
  - *Overall survival:* 95%
  - *Progression to TTTS:* 15%
  - Ultrasound scans every 1–2 weeks to monitor evolution
- *Stage 1:*
  - *Survival:* Overall 85%, at least one twin 90%
  - *Progression to stages 2–4:* 20%
  - Ultrasound scans every 1 week to monitor evolution
  - Endoscopic laser ablation of communicating placental vessels if progression to stages 2–4 or increasing polyhydramnios and shortening of cervical length.
- *Stages 2–4:*
  - *<28 weeks:* The best management is endoscopic laser ablation of communicating placental vessels; all communicating vessels should be ablated and the area between them should also be coagulated to achieve dichorionization of the placenta.
  - *≥28 weeks:* The best option is to deliver by cesarean section and the timing would depend on the Doppler findings in the umbilical artery and ductus venosus of both fetuses.
  - *Stage 2:* Survival overall 75%, at least one twin 85%.
  - *Stages 3 and 4:* Survival overall 60–70%, at least one twin 75–85%.
  - *Neurodevelopmental impairment in survivors:* 5–10%.

TAPS

- *Spontaneous:* 5% of monochorionic twins. Usually occurs >26 weeks' gestation.
- *After laser ablation of placental vessels:* 2–10% of monochorionic twins.
- Ultrasound diagnosis
- TAPS occurs due to a slow transfusion of blood from the donor to the recipient through few very small arteriovenous vascular anastomoses leading to highly discordant hemoglobin levels.
- There is no substantial difference between the twins in either size or amniotic fluid volume.
- The placenta of the anemic fetus looks thick and hyperechogenic, whereas that of the polycythemic fetus looks thin and translucent.
- The fetal middle cerebral artery peak systolic velocity (MCA-PSV) in the anemic fetus is increased (>1.5 multiples of median), whereas that in the polycythemic fetus it is decreased (<1 multiples of the normal median).
- The anemic fetus may have a dilated heart, tricuspid regurgitation, and ascites. The liver of the polycythemic fetus has a starry sky pattern due to diminished echogenicity of the liver parenchyma and an increased brightness of the portal venule walls.

Management

- *<26 weeks:* Endoscopic laser ablation of communicating placental vessels. Subsequently, scans every 1 week to monitor fetal growth, brain anatomy and MCA-PSV. Fetal brain MRI at ≥32 weeks' gestation should be considered for the diagnosis of neuronal migration disorders. If both babies are developing normally, vaginal delivery can be carried out at 37 weeks.
- *26–30 weeks:* Intrauterine blood transfusions to the anemic twin and exchange transfusion with Hartmann's solution for the polycythemic twin. Doppler assessment every 2–3 days because it may become necessary to undertake interventions every 3–4 days. Delivery by cesarean section at 30–32 weeks.
- *>30 weeks:* Delivery by cesarean section
- *Uncomplicated Monochorionic-diamniotic pregnancy:* Preferably between 36.0 and 37.0 weeks.
- *Uncomplicated Monochorionic-monoamniotic pregnancy:* Preferably between 32.0 and 32.6 weeks.
- Fetal lung maturation (betamethasone 12 mg/24 h 2 doses) and fetal neuroprotection ($MgSO_4$) should be administered prior to delivery by elective cesarean section.
- In twin or triplet pregnancies with a monochorionic component that are delivered before 34.0 weeks, fetal neuroprotection with $MgSO_4$ prior to birth is recommended, regardless of the mode of delivery.
- Neuroprotection will also be recommended in cases of monochorionic pregnancy and previous history of fetal surgery (cord occlusion, laser) if delivered before 34.0 weeks.

MC twins are associated with a 2- to 3-fold increase in the risk of malformations as compared with singletons and dichorionic twins, most of which are discordant, i.e., present in only one twin.

- There is a higher prevalence of congenital cardiac defects, which should be identified before deciding the type of therapy and counseling the parents.
- TTTS is associated with pulmonary stenosis/atresia in up to 10–15% of cases, normally in stage III onward but sometimes in earlier stages.
- Part of these cases will reverse during pregnancy or after birth, but up to 30% may persist postnatally.
- It may be very difficult or impossible to ascertain whether pulmonary stenosis/atresia is purely functional or anatomic, and this can only be seen with follow-up.
- Tricuspid regurgitation is a common finding in the recipient, but it does not modify prognosis when the severity staging is used, and therefore it is not used as a severity criterion.
- In the presence of a discordant fetal anomaly, the possibility of selective termination may be discussed with the parents.

Q6. Which are the common post treatment complications in MC?

Draft Recommendation:

- Most common posttreatment complications in monochorionic twin pregnancy include TAPS.
- *After laser ablation of placental vessels:* 2-10% of monochorionic twins.
- *Ultrasound diagnosis:*
    - TAPS occurs due to a slow transfusion of blood from the donor to the recipient through few very small arteriovenous vascular anastomoses leading to highly discordant hemoglobin levels.
    - There is no substantial difference between the twins in either size or amniotic fluid volume.
- The placenta of the anemic fetus looks thick and hyperechogenic, whereas that of the polycythemic fetus looks thin and translucent.
- The fetal middle cerebral artery peak systolic velocity (MCA PSV) in the anemic fetus is increased (>1.5 multiples of median), whereas that in the polycythemic fetus is decreased (<1 multiples of the normal median).
- The anemic fetus may have a dilated heart, tricuspid regurgitation and ascites. The liver of the polycythemic fetus has a starry sky pattern due to diminished echogenicity of the liver parenchyma and an increased brightness of the portal venule walls.

Q7. What are the best practices for coordinating care among the health care team?

Draft Recommendation:

- Counselling the patient
- Initial Assessment
- Explain Monochorionic Twin Pregnancies:
- Define Monochorionic Twins
- Clarify Differences
- Discuss Specific Risks and Complications
- Outline Monitoring and Management
- Educate on Symptoms and When to Seek Help
- Provide Emotional and Psychological Support
- Offer Educational Materials
- Regular Follow-Up and Communication

Coordinating the team*:*

- Multidisciplinary team approach
- Establish Clear Communication Channels
- Create Comprehensive Care Plans
- Ensure Coordination of Services
- Prioritize Preventive Care and Early Intervention:
- Document and Share Information Efficiently

Summary of evidence:

- All sonographers who undertake routine ultrasound scans during pregnancy must be trained to establish chorionicity and the correct labelling of twins.
- All sonographers who undertake midtrimester (18+0–20+6 weeks) and fetal growth scans of monochorionic twins should be made aware of the appearances of TTTS, sFGR and TAPS, and the need to refer patients on to specialist centres if such features present.
- Fetal medicine centres undertaking fetal therapy for relatively rare complications of monochorionic twins should have a minimum of two experienced operators and more than 15 cases per year(rolling 3-year average) to maximize perinatal outcomes and minimize long-term morbidity.

BIBLIOGRAPHY

1. Ponce J, Bennasar M, Crovetto F, Eixarch E, Martínez JM, Gratacós E. Monochorionic twin pregnancy: twin-to-twin transfusion syndrome (TTTS). [online] Available from https://fetalmedicinebarcelona.org/wp-content/uploads/2024/08/Guidelines_TTTS.pdf [Last accessed December, 2024]. Júlia Ponce, Mar Bennasar, Francesca Crovetto, Elisenda Eixarch, Josep Maria Martínez,Eduard Gratacós
2. Ponce J, Bennasar M, Martínez JM, Marimón E, Eixarch E, Gratacós E, et al. Monochorionic twin pregnancy: selective fetal growth restriction (sFGR). Júlia Ponce, Mar Bennasar, Josep Maria Martínez, Edda Marimón, Elisenda Eixarch, Eduard Gratacós[online] Available from https://fetalmedicinebarcelona.org/wp-content/uploads/2024/06/Guidelines-sFGR-MC.pdf [Last accessed December, 2024].
3. Rodgers KA, Baschat A, et al. ISUOG Practice Guidelines: role of ultrasound in twin pregnancy. Ultrasound Obstet Gynecol. 2016;47:247-63.
4. Ultrasound Obstet Gynecol. 2016;47:247-2-63. doi: 10.1002/uog.15821.

CHAPTER 6

Immunologically Positive Pregnancy

Seetha Pal

KEY QUESTIONS

1. Why is there a female predominance? Does pregnancy, parity, or other hormonal factors explain this?
2. Do we need to screen for such conditions in pregnancy?
3. How safe is it for the mother with autoimmune (AI) conditions to get pregnant, in acute and chronic phase?
4. Does the disease alter the course or outcome of pregnancy?
5. What are the risks of passage of maternal autoantibodies to the fetus?
6. Which autoimmune drugs are permissible in pregnancy?
7. What are the additional maternal and fetal surveillance required in these pregnancies?
8. What are the prophylactic measures to prevent adverse outcomes in the mother?
9. What are the new therapeutic and management approaches improve the pregnancy outcomes in women with autoimmune diseases?

Q1. Why is there a female predominance? Does pregnancy, parity, or other hormonal factors explain this?

Draft recommendations:

- The prevalence of autoimmune conditions is higher in women and is almost two-fold. As autoimmune conditions are more prevalent in women of reproductive age, they are the commonest preexisting conditions found in pregnancy.
- Parity per se does not have an effect on prevalence.

Summary of evidence: A Danish registry study reported a rise in prevalence from 3.7 to 15.8% between 1989 and 2013; a four- to eight-fold rise was demonstrated for the autoimmune diseases rheumatoid arthritis (from 0.1 to 0.73%), systemic lupus erythematosus (from 0.02 to 0.07%), chronic inflammatory bowel disease (from 0.3 to 1.09%), and multiple sclerosis (from 0.04 to 0.26%).

Q2. Do we need to screen for such conditions in pregnancy and what are the diagnostic features?

Draft recommendations:

- Though routine screening may not be cost effective in low-risk population, women with chronic medical disorders and previous bad obstetric outcome may benefit by screening for autoimmune conditions.

- Specific clinical and laboratory criteria have been identified for diagnosing primary antiphospholipid syndrome.

Summary of evidence: International consensus statement on an update of the classification criteria for definite APS syndrome 2006 has laid down specific clinical and laboratory criteria for diagnosing APS.

- One or more unexplained deaths of a morphologically normal fetus at or beyond the 10th week of gestation, *or*
- One or more premature births of a morphologically normal neonate before the 34th week of gestation because of eclampsia, severe preeclampsia, or recognized features of placental insufficiency, *or*
- Three or more unexplained consecutive spontaneous abortions before the 10th week of gestation with maternal anatomic or hormonal abnormalities and paternal and maternal chromosomal causes excluded.

The laboratory criteria are the presence of LA in plasma, medium, or high titers of aCL of the IgG or IgM isotypes (>40 GPL or MPL, or > the 99th percentile), or aβ2GPI of the IgG or IgM isotypes (in titer > the 99th percentile). All positive tests should be confirmed at least 12 weeks apart.

Q3. How safe is it for the mother with autoimmune (AI) conditions to get pregnant, in acute and chronic phase?

Draft recommendations:

- Symptoms of autoimmune conditions could improve, worsen, or remain unchanged in pregnancy and postpartum depending on her specific autoimmune condition.
- Generally, if the symptoms are well controlled and the disease is in remission phase, there is no contraindication to conceive.

Summary of evidence: Some conditions such as rheumatoid arthritis tend to improve in pregnancy while women with SLE can have exacerbation of symptoms and some tend to remain unchanged. Although the reasons for these differences are unclear, they have been linked to the complex immunological mechanism that occur in pregnancy.

American College of Rheumatology guideline recommends patients with known autoimmune diseases should not have active disease and should ideally be in remission phase before they embark on a pregnancy to prevent disease exacerbations in pregnancy.

Q4. Does the disease alter the course or outcome of pregnancy?

Draft recommendations: Many autoimmune conditions can have an adverse effect on maternal and fetal outcome and this can be attributed both to the condition itself and the medication that the patient is on.

Poorly controlled disease is associated with poor maternal outcomes like early onset preeclampsia and fetal effects can range from both early and late miscarriage, fetal growth restriction, preterm birth, and intrauterine fetal death.

Summary of evidence: EULAR guidelines state that:

- *SLE activity/flares (in the last 6–12 months or at conception):* Increased risk for (1) maternal disease activity (RR 2.1 for subsequent flare during pregnancy and puerperium); (2) hypertensive complications (OR 1.8 for PE); (3) fetal morbidity and mortality (OR 5.7 for pregnancy loss, 16 3.5 for IUGR17 6.5 for preterm delivery).
- *Lupus nephritis (history or active at conception):* Strong predictor of poor maternal (RR 9.0 for renal flare during/after pregnancy) and fetal outcome(s) (OR 7.3 for fetal loss and 18.9 for preterm delivery).
- *Serological (serum C3/C4, anti-dsDNA titers) activity:* Increased risk for maternal SLE flares during pregnancy (OR 5.3) and pregnancy loss
- *Previous adverse pregnancy outcome(s) APS:* Increased risk for pregnancy complications
- *History of vascular thrombosis APS:* Increased risk (ORs ranging 3.6–12.7) for pregnancy morbidity
- *aPL profile with SLE:* Strong predictor of adverse maternal and fetal outcomes, especially for patients with persistent moderate-to-high aPL titers, LA, and multiple aPL positivity (high-risk aPL profile).
- *APS:* High-risk aPL profile correlates with increased risk of maternal vascular thrombotic events during pregnancy (OR 12.1), (pre-)eclampsia (OR 2.3), APS-related pregnancy morbidity (OR 9.2), IUGR (OR 4.7), preterm birth.

Q5. What are the risks of passage of maternal autoantibodies to the fetus?

Draft recommendations:

- During normal pregnancy, there is a physiological transfer of immunoglobulins from the mother to the fetus, with the aim of providing essential protection during the first few months of life when neonatal humoral response is inefficient.
- Despite their clear benefit, in women with autoimmune conditions, the harmful antibodies can cross the placenta and cause fetal complications.
- The antibodies vary according to the autoimmune condition and can cause varied fetal effects.

Summary of evidence:

- *Thyroid receptor antibodies:* Transplacental passage of maternal thyroid receptor or antibodies in women with Graves' disease can cause neonatal goiter and hyperthyroidism. Sometimes the maternal antithyroid medication or thyroid blocking antibodies can cause hypothyroid goiter.

- *Anti Ro, Anti La antibodies:* Anti Ro and Anti La antibodies which were initially described in association with SLE and Sjogren's syndrome can be found with other autoimmune disorders such as mixed connective disorders or systemic sclerosis. Transplacental passage of these antibodies can cause neonatal lupus and complete AV block in the fetus which can occur in 2% of nulliparous women and 205 of women with previously affected fetus. This can be fatal in about 15% of fetuses, if complete heart block progresses to fetal hydrops.
- *ITP antibodies:* Patients with immune mediated thrombocytopenia can have IgG platelet specific antibodies that can induce fetal platelet destruction and neonatal thrombocytopenia and if severe, intracranial hemorrhage.
- *Anti-AChR antibodies:* Patients with myasthenia gravis have autoantibodies directed against the acetylcholine receptors and their transplacental passage can produce transient neonatal myasthenia gravis in 15% of cases. Sometimes, it may be involved in fetal arthrogryposis congenita.

Q6. Which autoimmune drugs are permissible in pregnancy?

Draft recommendations:

- Women with autoimmune conditions are usually on immune suppressive drugs and these can affect the fetus.
- Some drugs are not permissible in pregnancy and ideally women should be on stable regimen before conception and postpartum.
- In general, these medications can be considered in four categories:
    - Low risk in pregnancy
    - Low risk emerging therapies with developing evidence for use during pregnancy
    - Intermediate risk with little or no existing data on use in pregnancy, and
    - High-risk medications generally contraindicated in pregnancy
- Drugs such as hydroxychloroquine, oral glucocorticoids, azathioprine, cyclosporin-A and tacrolimus can be prescribed to prevent or manage flares during pregnancy and can be safely used in lactation too.

Summary of evidence: ACOG and EULAR guidelines state that most commonly prescribed drugs can be used safely in pregnancy but a few are strictly contraindicated. Decisions regarding medication should be individualized and taken in a multidisciplinary approach.

Drugs to be stopped before pregnancy (3–6 months before planned pregnancy)	***Drugs with insufficient data***	***Drugs permitted in pregnancy***
Methotrexate	Leflunomide	Steroids
Cyclophosphamide	Mepacrine	Hydroxychloroquine
Mycophenolate mofetil	Selective cox 2 inhibitors	Azathioprine, Cyclosporine
Warfarin (stopped when pregnancy test positive)	Statins	Tacrolimus, sulfasalazine, colchicine
		Iv immunoglobulin
		TNF alpha inhibitors

Q7. What are the additional maternal and fetal surveillance required in these pregnancies?

Draft recommendations:

- Women with autoimmune disorders should receive individual and inter disciplinary care prior to conception.
- Screening for malnutrition especially in women with inflammatory bowel disease should be done and corrected if needed.
- Baseline bloods, screening for asymptomatic bacteriuria, serological profile with complement levels relevant to the disorder.
- Multimodal screening for preeclampsia should be done in all the trimesters.
- Postnatal screening for relapse
- *Fetal screening:*
    - First trimester combined screening for aneuploidies, preeclampsia, FGR, and first trimester anomaly scan or NIPT with detailed scan.
    - Second trimester detailed anomaly scan with uterine artery Doppler assessment.
    - Fetal echocardiography
    - In women with Anti Ro and La antibodies, weekly assessment of fetal heart from 16 weeks.
    - Serial growth and doppler scans from 28 weeks onward every 4 weeks or otherwise depending on the severity of the condition.
    - Neonatal screening for heart block.

Summary of evidence: RCOG, ACOG, and EULAR guidelines recommend close monitoring of the mother to detect disease flares, complications and fetal monitoring to detect structural anomalies and growth restriction.

Q8. What are prophylactic measures to prevent adverse outcomes in the mother?

Draft recommendations:

- *Hydroxychloroquine* is recommended preconceptionally and throughout pregnancy for patients with SLE.

- For prevention of preeclampsia, (especially those with lupus nephritis or positive aPL) *low-dose aspirin (ideally 150 mg)* from 12 weeks of pregnancy
- In women with SLE-associated APS and primary APS, *combination treatment with LDA preconceptionally and low molecular weight heparin as soon as pregnancy test positive*
- Patients with APS and previous thrombosis should receive low-dose aspirin and full anticoagulation during pregnancy and 6 weeks postpartum.
- Supplementation with *calcium, vitamin D,* and *folic acid* should be offered as in the general population.

Summary of evidence: EULAR, ACOG, RCOG, and ESHRE all endorse the use of HCQs, aspirin, and low-molecular weight heparin to reduce adverse maternal and fetal outcome. Maternal use of HCQ and corticosteroids help in disease suppression in pregnancy and maternal HCQ use may be associated with reduced rates of cardiac manifestations in the newborn.

Q9. What are the new therapeutic approaches improving the pregnancy outcomes in women with autoimmune diseases?

Draft recommendations:

- Newer classes of immunomodulating medications are being used in clinical practice due to their disease-modifying effects.
- Tumor necrosis factor-α inhibitor drugs such as infliximab, etanercept, adalimumab, certolizumab, and golimumab can be used as maintenance medications.
- *Biologicals:* These are monoclonal antibodies that interfere with immune response.

Summary of evidence: Limited evidence as of now regarding the use of newer immunomodulating drugs. The risk of using certain biological agents in pregnancy is not from proven teratogenicity but is due to unknown long-term safety for the fetus. Considering the lack of data, most authors recommend discontinuation of therapy as soon as pregnancy is diagnosed.

BIBLIOGRAPHY

1. ACOG Committee Opinion No. 776: Immune Modulating Therapies in Pregnancy and Lactation. Obstet Gynecol. 2019;133(4):e287-95.
2. Andreoli L, Bertsias GK, Agmon-Levin N, et al. EULAR recommendations for women's health and the management of family planning, assisted reproduction, pregnancy and menopause in patients with systemic lupus erythematosus and/or antiphospholipid syndrome. Ann Rheumat Dis. 2017;76:476-85.
3. ESHRE Guideline Group on RPL; Bender Atik R, Christiansen OB, et al. ESHRE guideline: recurrent pregnancy loss: an update in 2022. Hum Reprod Open. 2023;2023(1): hoad002.
4. Singh M, Wambua S, Lee SI, et al. Autoimmune diseases and adverse pregnancy outcomes: an umbrella review. BMC Med. 2024;94.

7

CHAPTER

Fetal Teratogens

Chitra Andrew

INTRODUCTION

KEY QUESTIONS

1. Which are the common fetal teratogens which should be ideally counseled regarding effective contraception and role of preconception counseling?
2. What should be counseled when the exposure has occurred regarding the possible lethal or resultant long-term abnormalities which may occur as a result of teratogens?
3. What is effect of X-ray exposure on the fetus and the advice based on exposure?
4. What are the effects of medication for chronic illness? What are the acceptable doses and recommendations for surveillance?
5. What are the effects of habit-related consumption of substances? What are the acceptable doses and recommendations for surveillance?
6. What are the effects of infections? What are the recommendations for surveillance?

Q1. Which are the common fetal teratogens which should be ideally counseled regarding effective contraception and role of preconception counseling?

Draft recommendations:

- Exposure to all teratogens should ideally be avoided in pregnancy and in the periconceptional period as they cause about 5% of anomalies and may have long-term effects on cognition and physical development.
- Anything that a person ingests or is exposed to, which is a known cause of fetal abnormalities is a teratogen.
- Some medicines, chemicals (mercury, lead), and certain infections (CMV, Zika, and toxoplasmosis) and radiation are examples of teratogens which should ideally be avoided during pregnancy.
- The exposure to these medications either as treatment of chronic conditions or as an investigatory modality should be carefully assessed with regard to dose and duration of exposure.

Summary of evidence: The American college of Obstetrics and Gynecology (ACOG) (2014) Preconception and interconception care documents the need for accurate awareness of pregnancy prior to starting certain medications in women, additionally pre-conceptional counselling, adequate contraception and reduction or modification of the drug may be considered.

Evidence gap: Due to the nature of the condition, rarity of the results of exposure, and the ethical difficulties surrounding exposure to pregnant women, there is paucity of evidence on safety of medications. This translates into avoidance of essential drugs in certain conditions. There is a need for more studies to reassure regarding safety in this regard. Maintaining a database of the adverse effects of known exposures will give additional relevant information.

Q2. What should be counseled when the exposure has occurred regarding the possible lethal or resultant long-term abnormalities which may occur as a result of teratogens?

Draft recommendations:

- Important factors such as gestational age of the fetus at exposure, dose of the drug, and any genetic factors influencing metabolism of the drug which would increase the teratogenic risk should be enquired and documented.
- In order to determine the extent of possible damage due to the teratogen, the factors which are important include the chemical and duration of exposure.

Summary of evidence: Multiple reviews and meta-analyses are published regarding medications, chemicals, and viruses. These summarize the effect and neonatal manifestations of the conditions.

Evidence gap: Despite multiple studies, there is lack of knowledge of the dose exposure in many instances of chemical and toxin exposure, (e.g., mercury, cadmium, and lead poisoning) where timing and dose are difficult to study in real life circumstance. This will require further study.

Q3. What is the effect of X-ray exposure on the fetus and the advice based on exposure?

Draft recommendations:

- Determining the presence of pregnancy prior to radiation exposure is important because exposure to irradiation has a dose-related effect on the fetus which is also altered by the gestational age at exposure.
- As many exposures occur inadvertently as the woman may be unaware that she is pregnant or is in very early pregnancy, enquiry regarding last menstrual period and use of contraception is essential.
- In cases of inadvertent exposure to radiation, counseling should be based on the modality used (e.g., computed tomography or contrast), gestational age at exposure and duration of exposure.
- Additionally, all needed investigations including imaging should not be withheld from the woman, due to a possible pregnancy or as the woman is breastfeeding; as this can lead to misdiagnosis or delay in diagnosis of a condition which is detrimental to the health of the woman.

Summary of evidence: The ACOG committee opinion, No. 723, October 2017, (Revalidated 2021), provides a clear guideline on the doses of exposure that is likely to cause harm to the fetus.

The risk to a fetus is dependent on the gestational age at exposure and the dose of radiation. High doses of irradiation are known to cause fetal growth restriction, intellectual disability, and microcephaly. The greatest risk may be between 8 and 15 weeks and the dose of 60–310 mGy (milli-Gray) as a minimum threshold. This can be compared to the dose exposure to the fetus in common tests—e.g., abdominal X-ray = 0.1–3 mGy, intravenous pyelogram 5-10 mGy, chest X-ray two views = 0.0005–0.01 mGy.

Evidence gap: Use of gadolinium as contrast in MRI has been studies extensively but due to the lack of proper control group and the rarity of inflammatory and rheumatic conditions, the safety of gadolinium contrast in pregnancy requires further evaluation.

Q4. What are the effects of medication for chronic illness? What are the acceptable doses and recommendations for surveillance?

Draft recommendations:

- Depending on the nature and requirement for medications, women with chronic medical illnesses requiring medicines should be counseled preconceptionally and adequate contraception discussed if required.
- If a pregnancy is planned, a discussion with the concerned specialist to alter, reduce or stop the drug should be performed at an appropriate time.
- In case of an unplanned pregnancy, the medication should be carefully reviewed and consultations made with specialists regarding the need for dose alteration, change of medication or discontinuation of medication.
- Due care must be taken to warn women not to stop medications without medical advice as this may be potentially dangerous to the woman (e.g., anticonvulsants, bronchodilators, antihypertensives, etc.)
- In some cases, a time period of contraception can be advised based on the condition to allow time for the excretion of the teratogen, e.g., radioactive iodine.

Summary of evidence: The green top guideline No. 68 discusses the role of anti-epileptic medication and the dangers of discontinuing medication. Similarly, the NICE guideline CG192 antenatal and postnatal mental health: Clinical management and service guidance discusses medications used in mental illness.

Evidence gap: Newer and more effective medications are added to the armamentarium of treatment and it is vital that the potential teratogenicity of these drugs are studied to be able to use these medications safely.

Here we summarize a few commonly used medications and the teratogenic effects of the same.

Medications used for treatment and their teratogenic effects are given here in tabulated form.

Anticonvulsant medications	***Epilepsy during pregnancy can cause falls, sudden unexplained death, and status epilepticus. Therefore, it is not recommended to stop medications without specialist advice.***		
Teratogen	***Physical features***	***Disabilities***	***Recommendation***
Valproic acid	Cranofacial anomalies: Midface hypoplasia, epicanthal folds, short nose, broad nasal bridge, thin upper lip, thick lower lip, micrognathia, cardiac anomalies (VSD, coarctation aorta)	Long-term effects include: reduced cognitive ability, autism, and attention-deficit /hyperactivity disorder	RCOG guidelines suggest that valproic acid be avoided in women of child bearing age
Carbamazepine	Upslanting palpebral fissures, a long philtrum, and nail hypoplasia, as well as growth deficiency and microcephaly		Can be used as the incidence of anomalies is low
Lamotrigine			Less anomalies reported for this mediation
Levetiracetam			Less anomalies reported for this mediation
Immunosuppressive agents			
Mycophenolate mofetil		Microtia or anotia, oral clefts, and conotruncal heart defects	3 months of medication avoidance prior to conception
Corticosteroids	Inhaled corticosteroids (asthma), topical preparations		No evidence of increased anomalies
	Systemic prednisone, prednisolone	>5/1,000—orofacial clefts, fetal growth restriction–may be due to underlying cause, dose related	Dose-related risk and low incidence of anomalies

Contd...

Contd...

Anticonvulsant medications	***Epilepsy during pregnancy can cause falls, sudden unexplained death, and status epilepticus. Therefore, it is not recommended to stop medications without specialist advice.***		
Teratogen	***Physical features***	***Disabilities***	***Recommendation***
Folate antagonist			
Methotrexate		Severe lack of calvarial ossification, hypoplastic supraorbital ridges, small and low-set ears, micrognathia, limb abnormalities, developmental delay	Contraception for 3–12 months depending on the dose given
Vitamin K antagonists	Fetal warfarin syndrome		
Warfarin and phenindione	Intellectual disability, microcephaly, hydrocephalus, Dandy–Walker malformation, or agenesis of the corpus callosum, and eye defects such as optic atrophy or cataracts	Nasal hypoplasia, stippled epiphyses visible on radiographs, and growth restriction	
Angiotensin I—converting enzyme (ACE) inhibitor (e.g., enalapril) or angiotensin II receptor antagonist (ARB; e.g., losartan)	Fetal hypotension with consequent hypoperfusion and oligohydramnios	• Renal tubular dysplasia, oligohydramnios, hypocalvarium • Fetal renal failure and oligohydramnios, leading to fetal growth restriction, calvarial hypoplasia, joint contractures, and pulmonary hypoplasia	Stop the medicine with specialist consultation at the earliest and substitute
Oral isotretinoin	Rapid systemic absorption	20% risk of brain, conotruncal heart, ear, and thymus malformations, and an even higher risk of intellectual disability in liveborn children	
Topical tretinoin	Poorly absorbed through the skin	Is not associated with an increased risk of the same pattern of adverse effects	

Q5. What are the effects of habit-related consumption of substances? What are the acceptable doses and recommendations for surveillance?

Draft recommendation:

- In case of substance misuse (e.g., alcohol, recreational drugs) where compliance with deaddiction services may be the issue, adequate counseling will be required based on the specific condition and gestational age.
- When the teratogenic agent is related to substance misuse, counseling toward lifestyle modification preferably preconception but at the least from booking visit is recommended.
- Women who are pregnant should be made aware of the teratogenic effects of alcohol, recreational drugs and smoking (including second hand smoke) and adequate support provided to modify lifestyle and protect the fetus and newborn.
- In some circumstances, substitution and detoxification and other aid may be required to reduce high-risk behavior.

Summary of evidence: The NICE guideline CG 110, pregnancy and complex social factors: A model for service provision for pregnant women with complex social factors details the challenges face by the women and care providers. Social factors and peer support play a large role in sustaining behavior modification.

Evidence gap: Studies and longitudinal follow-up have failed to show a consistent permanent lifestyle change in women with various addictions and the optimal combination of methods to prove effective in this regard has yet to be discovered.

Teratogen	*Condition*	*Features*	*Dose/ recommendation*
Alcohol	Fetal alcohol syndrome	Abnormal facies, long philtrum, learning difficulties, conotruncal anomalies, behavioral issues, difficulty in perception	No dose is safe in pregnancy
Smoking	Causes degenerative changes in the placenta	• Fetal growth restriction, preterm labor, miscarriage • *Anomalies:* cardiovascular, musculoskeletal, and gastroschisis	
Cocaine marijuana heroin	Neonatal abstinence syndrome	• Crying, sweating, poor feeds = withdrawal symptoms • Cocaine is a risk factor for abruption	
Opioids		Preterm labor, fetal growth restriction, reduced fetal heart rate, and fetal activity	No increase in congenital anomalies

Q6. What are the effects of infections? What are the recommendations for surveillance?

Draft recommendations:

- Women who are planning pregnancy or are pregnant already should be counseled regarding the need for avoidance of contact with those with infections.
- If exposure to an infection should occur they should report to their doctor and promptly be sent to a relevant specialist for further investigations as required.
- Fetal surveillance in the form of serial ultrasound to assess growth and development of any structural abnormalities should be performed by fetal medicine specialists.
- Antiviral or other relevant medications will have to be commenced.
- In selected cases, based on the timing of the exposure and nature of the infection, direct testing by amniocentesis for viral polymerase chain reaction (PCR) testing can be offered.
- Termination of pregnancy may be an option based on the gestational age and the results of investigations.

Summary of evidence: Chicken pox in pregnancy and the investigations are discussed in detail in Green top guideline no 13 from RCOG. This details the prevention, postexposure prophylaxis, and treatment of women with varicella exposure. The British Medical Bulletin 2017, discusses the effects of Zika and prevention, contraception, and ultrasound monitoring for microcephaly in women who are affected. A recent review of all evidence on guidelines pertaining to cytomegalovirus states that routine serological testing is not indicated in pregnancy. The review also stated that valaciclovir as an intervention lacked data.

Evidence gap: Since the incidence of infections in pregnancy is often not proved and followed-up, development of adequate testing modalities, vaccination and prevention of exposure, and contraception following exposure are areas which need further study.

Viral infections causing teratogenicity.

Virus	*Fetal effects*	*Surveillance*	
Zika virus	Microcephaly, cerebral calcifications, atrophy of the cerebellum, and brainstem	Serial growth and fetal neurosonography	
Rubella virus	Cataract, deafness, cardiac defects, anemia, and hepatosplenomegaly	Fetal growth restriction, fetal anemia, on MCA Doppler	Prevention by vaccination of school-age girls and boys

Contd...

Contd...

Virus	***Fetal effects***	***Surveillance***	
			• May be detected only at birth • Maternal serology IgG, IgM, if suspected, amniotic fluid for viral PCR
Parvovirus	Fetal anemia, hydrops, and fetal death	Fetal anemia on MCA Doppler	• Fetal intrauterine blood, transfusion. • No antiviral or vaccine available
Cytomega-lovirus	Fetal growth restriction, hepatosplenomegaly, pneumonia, pancytopenia		Antiviral ganciclovir can be offered if the parents elect to continue the pregnancy
Varicella Zoster	Reactivation of the virus and invasion of the placenta is thought to be the cause of infection	CNS: Cortical atrophy, microcephaly, chorioretinitis	About 2% of pregnancies affected in first trimester exposure
	Women developing chicken pox in early pregnancy should be referred to a fetal medicine center at 16–20 weeks or 5 weeks after infection. Amniocentesis has a strong negative predictive value but a weak positive predictive value. So, the pros and cons of direct testing have to be explained to the couple		
	If maternal infection occurs in the last 4 weeks of pregnancy, a planned delivery should normally be avoided for at least 7 days after the onset of the maternal rash to allow for the passive transfer of antibodies from mother to child. This is only if provided that continuing the pregnancy does not pose any additional risks to the mother or baby		

BIBLIOGRAPHY

1. ACOG committee opinion, No. 723. (2017). Diagnostic imaging during pregnancy and lactation. [online] Available from https://www.acog.org/clinical/clinical-guidance/committee-opinion/articles/2017/10/guidelines-for-diagnostic-imaging-during-pregnancy-and-lactation [Last accessed November, 2024].
2. American college of obstetrics and Gynecology. (2014). Preconception and interconception care, in guidelines for Women's care, a resource manual. [online] Available from https://www.acog.org/clinical/clinical-guidance/committee-opinion/articles/2019/01/prepregnancy-counseling [Last accessed November, 2024].

3. Green top guideline No. 13. (2015). Chicken pox in pregnancy. [online] Available from https://www.rcog.org.uk/guidance/browse-all-guidance/green-top-guidelines/chickenpox-in-pregnancy-green-top-guideline-no-13/ [Last accessed November, 2024].
4. Green top guideline No. 68. (2016). Epilepsy in pregnancy. [online] Available from https://www.rcog.org.uk/guidance/browse-all-guidance/green-top-guidelines/epilepsy-in-pregnancy-green-top-guideline-no-68/[Last accessed November, 2024].
5. Morrison JO. Opioid misuse in pregnancy TOG Obstet Gynaecol. 2022;24(2):85-150.
6. Xie M, Tripathi T, Holmes NE, et al. Serological screening for cytomegalovirus during pregnancy: A systematic review of clinical practice guidelines and consensus statements. Prenat Diagn. 2023;43(7):959-67.

8

CHAPTER

Intrauterine Fetal Demise

Manisha Madhai Beck, Sandhya Singh

INTRODUCTION

KEY QUESTIONS

1. How is stillbirth defined and classified?
2. What is the burden of the problem?
3. How is diagnosis of IUFD made? How and what do you tell the parents when diagnosis is confirmed?
4. What tests should be recommended to investigate IUFD?
5. How should pregnancy be terminated/labor induced following diagnosis of IUFD?
6. What are the risk factors and common causes of IUFD in the low- and middle-income countries?
7. What counseling should be offered to the couple regarding subsequent pregnancies?

Q1. How is stillbirth defined and classified?

Draft recommendations: Fetal demise or intrauterine fetal demise (IUFD) is defined as death of a fetus prior to the complete expulsion or its extraction from its mother of products of conception, at any gestational age. Stillbirth is defined as the delivery of a fetus, with no signs of life such as breathing, heartbeat, cord pulsations, or definitive movement of voluntary muscles.

WHO has recommended the use of the ICD PM classification for stillbirths.

Classification of IUFD:

- *Based on gestational age*
  - *Early fetal death:* Fetal demise between 20 and 27 weeks
  - *Late fetal death:* IUFD between 28 and 36 weeks
  - *Term IUFD:* After 37 weeks
- *Based on timing of IUFD:*
  - *Fresh stillbirth or intrapartum stillbirth:* These are cases where fetal demise occurs after the onset of labor and within <12 hours of delivery. There are no fetal skin changes, and no other signs of maceration. This category excludes severe lethal congenital abnormalities.
  - *Macerated stillbirth or antepartum stillbirth:* Fetal demise occurs in the antepartum period, and fetus is retained in uterus after its demise, leading to characteristic macerated look with skin discoloration or darkening, redness, peeling, and breakdown, at birth.

Summary of evidence: As per Royal College of Obstetricians and Gynaecologists (RCOG) guidelines and World Health Organization (WHO) stillbirth is defined after ≥24 weeks (and/or 500 g) whereas in US and India, cutoff is taken as ≥20 weeks (and/or 350 g) and ≥28 weeks (and/or 1,000 g), respectively.

For comparison across the countries, WHO recommends a cutoff for defining stillbirth as: Gestational age ≥28 weeks or fetal weight ≥1,000 g or crown heel length ≥35 cm.

Evidence gap: The period of viability varies across the world. Although, India considers 28 weeks as cutoff for viability, as per the Stillbirth Surveillance guidelines released by MoHFW, stillbirths will be reported after 20 weeks.

The WHO recommends that ICD 10 classification for all diseases including stillbirths but the variation in application of ICD10 to stillbirths is limited by the comparability of cause of stillbirths across different settings—hence the ICD PM classification is recommended.

Q2. What is the burden of the problem?

Draft recommendations: The IUFD is usually an unexpected event in pregnancy and clinicians need to be aware of facts while counseling patients. It is known that every day, there are 7,177 stillbirths worldwide. In India alone, there are 1,622 stillbirths per day, amounting to 592,070 stillbirths annually in the country.

Summary of evidence: As per Government of India (GOI) Operational guidelines for establishing Sentinel Stillbirth Surveillance system, out of a total of 2.65 million stillbirths occurring globally every year, 45% are intrapartum, while 55% occur antepartum (before the onset of labor).

India's Newborn Action Plan (INAP) outlines the Ministry of Health and Family Welfare's (MOHFW) vision and goal to end preventable stillbirths, aiming to achieve a "Single Digit Stillbirth Rate" (SBR) by 2030.

Evidence gap: The statistics are dependent on available data but considering that there are gaps in reporting and data collection, the actual numbers may be different.

Q3. How do you diagnose IUFD and counsel the couple?

Draft recommendations:

- Diagnosis of IUFD is made when there is absence of fetal cardiac activity on 2D USG as a good practice point, this diagnosis should preferably be confirmed by two doctors if possible.
- It would not be prudent to diagnose an IUFD on based on fetal auscultation or CTG alone.
- The pregnant woman should be counseled about this incident in a sensitive manner preferably with her husband/family members together

or as per her wishes. This counseling should ideally be handled by a senior consultant or the senior most team member in pressing circumstances.

- Parents should be given time to grieve and understand the implications of diagnosis. Wherever feasible (where there is no immediate risks to mother such as chorioamnionitis, preeclampsia, etc.), counseling maybe done in more than one sitting.
- Need for further evaluation, both maternal and fetal, should be emphasized. However, parental choices should be respected.
- Empathetic approach and continuity of care giving are important aspects.
- Psychological support should be offered to all couples with diagnosis of IUFD.

Summary of evidence: The RCOG GTG no 55 on the work up of late IUFD and stillbirths summarizes evidence-based recommendations and good practice points in this topic.

Evidence gap: There are no "definite" evidence-based recommendations for many of the practices mentioned here due to the individuality and delicate nature of this situation. However, these recommendations appear reasonable in daily clinical situation and may be accepted as "good practice points".

Q4. What tests should be recommended to investigate IUFD?

Draft recommendations

- Importance of maternal; fetal and placental evaluation should be emphasized.
- Parents must be counseled that despite extensive evaluation, a cause may not be found in up to half of the cases.
- Parental choices and religious beliefs should be respected while investigations for IUFD.

Tests for maternal wellbeing:

- *Hematology*—complete blood count; ABO and Rh typing, coagulation profile
- *Biochemistry*—C reactive protein (CRP)

Tests to determine cause and risk of recurrence:

- *Maternal testing*
  - HbA1c
  - Indirect Coomb's test
  - Red cell antibodies (in cases of fetal hydrops)
  - Thrombophilia screening including APLA profile—FGR or placental disease or history of personal or family history of thrombosis.
  - Anticardiolipin Ab; lupus anticoagulant; IgM and IgG beta 2 glycoprotein

  - TORCH including parvovirus serology (suspected maternal infection); VDRL
  - Culture and sensitivity
  - Blood, urine, high vaginal swabs; rectovaginal swabs to rule out GBS infection.
  - Thyroid function tests
  - Kleihauer Betke test (suspected fetomaternal hemorrhage)
  - Anti Ro and Anti La Ab—if hydrops or endomyocardial fibroelastosis or AV node calcification seen on USG.
  - Serum bile acid—if symptoms suggestive of cholestasis.
  - Parental blood karyotyping—if fetal unbalanced translocation or if fetal genetic testing fails and history of and postmortem suggestive of aneuploidy/RPL or recurrent IUFD.
- Gross examination of the fetus and placenta
- Special fetal testing
  - Fetal autopsy after consent
  - Infantogram
  - Fetal tissue for karyotyping/CMA/DNA storage
- Placental testing—gross and HPE: If parents decline autopsy, less invasive tests such as gross examination by a perinatal pathologist; photos; infantograms; fetal MRI or even USG maybe offered to find answers to cause of IUFD.

Summary of evidence: A descriptive review of major guidelines (Tsakiridis et al.—2022) has outlined all the tests and investigations in the management of stillbirth.

Evidence gap: There are no "definite" evidence-based recommendations for many of the practices mentioned here due to the individuality and delicate nature of this situation. However, these recommendations appear reasonable in daily clinical situation and may be accepted as "good practice points".

Q5. How should pregnancy be terminated/labor induced following diagnosis of IUFD?

Draft recommendations:

- Once the diagnosis of IUFD is confirmed, termination of pregnancy should be offered to the couple.
- Expectant management may be offered in cases where woman's life is not in danger.
- For termination of pregnancy in unscarred uterus, mifepristone and PGE1 combination is used. The dosage and frequency of dosing of PGE1 varies based on gestational age.

- For scarred uterus, oral mifepristone alone or in combination with mechanical methods such as Foley's catheter are recommended.
- Vaginal route of delivery is preferred, even in cases of previous 1 or 2 LSCS women with >2 LSCS should be offered hysterotomy/LSCS for delivery.

Treatment protocol in women with IUFD and unscarred uteruses. As per Federation of International Societies of Obstetricians and Gynaecologists (FIGO) 2023 guidelines:

Gestational Age ≤24 weeks
Mifepristone 200 mg + Misoprostol 400 µg 3–4 hourly PV/SL/BU till expulsion.

Gestational age 25–27 weeks
Mifepristone 200 mg + Misoprostol 200 µg 4 hourly PV/SL/BU till expulsion.

Gestational age ≥28 weeks
Mifepristone 200 mg + Misoprostol 25–50 µg 4 hourly PV/SL/BU till expulsion.
or
Misoprostol 25–50 µg 2 hourly PO.

In women with previous LSCS, RCOG guidelines recommend oral mifepristone alone (200 mg thrice daily for 2 days) without use of prostaglandins. Alternatively, mechanical methods such as transcervical Foley's bulb may be used.

As per FIGO guidelines, PGE 1 is safe in pregnancies with previous LSCS where gestational age is <28 weeks.

Summary of evidence: The Federation of International Societies of Obstetricians and Gynaecologists (FIGO) 2023 guidelines, ACOG and the RCOG have given recommendations for IOL in unscarred uterus with few suggestions for scarred uteruses.

Evidence gap: While there are several guidelines outlining treatment protocols in women with unscarred uterus, there are few guidelines for those with previous LSCS/uterine surgery.

Q6. What are the risk factors and common causes of IUFD in the low and middle income countries?

Draft recommendations

Maternal risk factors include:

- Age
- BMI >30 kg/m^2
- *Medical comorbidities:* Diabetes; hypertension; SLE; chronic renal disease
- *Obstetric complications:* Cholestasis of pregnancy
- Maternal infections such as syphilis; TORCH
- *Maternal exposure to drugs:* Cocaine; alcohol
- *Bad obstetric history:* Previous stillbirth

- Post-term pregnancy
- *Family history:* Arrhythmias or sudden infant deaths

Fetal risk factors:
- Multiple gestation
- Fetal growth restriction
- Fetal infections
- Fetomaternal hemorrhage
- Fetal anomalies

Placental risk factors:
- Uteroplacental insufficiency
- Abnormal cord insertion: Velamentous; marginal
- Placental tumors: Chorioangioma.

Causes of IUFD vary across the globe. While in the LMIC setting, most common causes include intrapartum causes and hypertensive disorders, in developed world, maternal medical conditions and genetic abnormalities are most common.

Summary of evidence: According to the Stillbirth Collaborative Research Network study, risk factors identifiable at the beginning of pregnancy only account for a small portion of stillbirth risk. Previous stillbirth or pregnancy loss due to preterm birth or fetal growth restriction are among the few factors that have shown predictive value. Women who have experienced an unexplained stillbirth before are at a higher risk of experiencing it again.

Evidence gap: Most of the IUFD occur in women with no identifiable risk factors. Previous pregnancy loss due to FGR/uteroplacental insufficiency is one of the clearly identified risk factors for subsequent stillbirths.

Q7. What counseling should be offered to the couple regarding subsequent pregnancies?

Draft recommendations:
- The couple should be seen in the clinic after 6–8 weeks of delivery, for further counseling, with all the reports. The recurrence risk depends upon the cause for IUFD. Prevention strategies for subsequent pregnancies also depend upon the etiological cause of IUFD.
- Recurrence risk of IUFD in subsequent pregnancy depends upon the cause of IUFD. Causes such as uteroplacental insufficiency are likely to recur in comparison to fetomaternal hemorrhage; intrauterine infections which are unlikely to recur.
- In cases of uteroplacental insufficiency, low dose aspirin ± heparin is given in next pregnancy, depending on whether APLA is present.

- Serial fetal growth assessment with Dopplers should be done after 28 weeks in all cases with previous stillbirths till delivery.
- Intrapartum causes are mostly preventable and can be prevented by adhering to institutional delivery.
- Timing and mode of delivery in subsequent pregnancy is also important.
- Care plan for subsequent pregnancy, labor, and delivery should be clearly documented in the clinical notes.

Summary of evidence: Most major academic bodies and databases (Cochrane, ACOG, RCOG, FIGO, Stillbirth society of India) have provided best practice recommendations regarding care for couples having suffered a stillbirth with the aim to manage the current pregnancy and work up for the cause to prevent recurrence.

Evidence gap: Most recommendations regarding management of pregnancy following stillbirths as stated earlier are based on clinical practice points rather than Grade A evidence because of the obvious difficulties in generating such evidence.

BIBLIOGRAPHY

1. ACOG Practice Bulletin No 10. (2020). Management of stillbirth. [online] Available from https://www.acog.org/clinical/clinical-guidance/obstetric-care-consensus/articles/2020/03/management-of-stillbirth [Last accessed November, 2024].
2. Boyle A, Preslar JP, Hogue CJ, et al. Route of delivery in women with stillbirth: results from the stillbirth collaborative research network. Obstet Gynecol. 2017;129(4):693-8.
3. figo.org. FIGO Mifepristone and Misoprostol dosing charts 2023. [online] Available from https://www.figo.org/sites/default/files/2023-10/Mifepristone%20%26%20Misoprostol%20Dosing%20Chart%202023.pdf [Last accessed November, 2024].
4. GOI. Operational Guidelines for Establishing Sentinel Stillbirth Surveillance System. [online] Available from https://nhm.gov.in/images/pdf/programmes/RBSK/Operational_Guidelines/Operational_Guidelines_for_establishing_Sentinel_Stillbirth_Surveillance_System.pdf [Last accessed November, 2024].
5. Khong TY, Mooney EE, Ariel I, et al. Sampling and definitions of placental lesions: Amsterdam placental workshop group consensus statement. Archives of pathology and laboratory medicine. 2016;140(7):698-713.
6. Lamont K, Scott N W, Jones G T, et al. Risk of recurrent stillbirth: systematic review and meta-analysis. BMJ. 2015;350:h3080.
7. Mohanasundari SK, Padmaja A. National Health Mission (NHM) and India Newborn Action Plan (INAP) Services in Newborn Health-An Overview. Int J Adv Nurs Manag. 2019;7(4):366-70.
8. RCOG Green Top guidelines No.55. Late intrauterine fetal death and stillbirth. [online] Available from https://www.rcog.org.uk/guidance/

browse-all-guidance/green-top-guidelines/care-of-late-intrauterine-fetal-death-and-stillbirth-green-top-guideline-no-55/ [Last accessed November, 2024].

9. Reinebrant HE, Leisher SH, Coory M, et al. Making stillbirths visible: a systematic review of globally reported causes of stillbirth. BJOG. 2018;125(2):212-24.
10. Sharma B, Siwatch S, Kakkar N, et al. Classifying stillbirths in a tertiary care hospital of India: International Classification of Disease-perinatal Mortality [ICD-PM] versus cause of death-associated condition [CODAC] system. J Obstet Gynaecol. 2021;41(2):229-33.
11. Stillbirth society of India. Consensus Statement 2023 for Evaluation after Stillbirth. [online] Available from https://stillbirthindia.org/Consensus.aspx [Last accessed November, 2024].
12. The Perinatal Society of Australia and New Zealand. Clinical practice Guidelines for perinatal mortality audit. [online] Available from https://sanda.psanz.com.au/assets/Uploads/Section-1-Version-2.2-April-2009.pdf [Last accessed November, 2024].
13. Tsakiridis I, Giouleka S, Mamopoulos A, et al. Investigation and management of stillbirth: a descriptive review of major guidelines. Journal of perinatal medicine. 2022;50(6):796-813.
14. Wojcieszek AM, Shepherd E, Middleton P, et al. Care prior to and during subsequent pregnancies following stillbirth for improving outcomes. Cochrane Database Syst Rev. 2018;12(12):CD012203.

CHAPTER 9

Fetal Surveillance and Antenatal Counseling for Surgically Correctable Defects

Rachna Gupta

KEY QUESTIONS

1. How to approach and counsel couple when fetal anomaly is detected?
2. What are the conditions that determine further testing or termination of pregnancy?
3. Which defects have less surgery-related mortality and a good quality of life postsurgical correction?
4. Which defects are at high risk or premature births and in need in-utero transfer to a higher/tertiary care center?
5. What are the defects in which prognosis depends not only on the defect but the changes caused by it?
6. Is the prognosis different in fetuses with cardiac defects?

Q1. How do you approach and counsel a couple when fetal anomaly is detected?

Draft recommendations:

- When a defect is identified in the developing fetus during pregnancy, caregivers need to approach the woman and the family with compassion and evidence-based facts for further counseling and management of the pregnancy.
- It is important to understand that defects diagnosed during pregnancy evolve with advancing gestational age which will have a bearing on the outcome. A one-point examination may not be enough to guide the prognostication.
- If the defect is deemed surgically correctable, serial follow-up by ultrasound, and counseling by a multidisciplinary team are important. This helps in accurate diagnosis of the underlying condition, prognostication, decision-making by the parents, and optimizing the outcome.
- The involvement of obstetrician, fetal medicine specialist, radiologist, pediatric surgeon and/or pediatric cardiologist, geneticist, neonatologist, psychologist, and social worker is important in counseling the family.
- Every case needs an individualized approach with the help of multidisciplinary team meetings. Counseling needs adequate time

and a compassionate approach, keeping in mind the parents' and families' thought processes, and needs, and addressing their concerns respectfully. Most importantly, termination is not the answer for structural defects.

Q2. What are the conditions that determine further testing or termination of pregnancy?

Draft recommendations:

- *The decision on whether to continue the pregnancy or not depends on various factors:*
  - Type and severity of the defect
  - Single/multiple organ involvement
  - System involved-brain/cardiac/face/thorax/abdomen/limbs/spine
  - Association with chromosomal or genetic abnormalities
  - Availability of infrastructure for neonatal surgery
  - Whether place and mode of delivery will be affected by the defect
  - Surgical cure rate
  - Number of surgeries required
  - Residual morbidity or quality of life after surgical repair
  - Cosmetic appearance after surgery
  - Religious or personal beliefs
  - Costs involved
  - Previous obstetric history
  - Method of conception
  - Gestational age at diagnosis
  - Law of the land
  - Singleton/multiple pregnancy; chorionicity
  - Involvement of trained personnel in counselling and management—pediatric surgery team, psychological support, and social support
- *Defects with a higher association with chromosomal or genetic abnormalities needing invasive tests (the list is not comprehensive and each case merits genetic counseling):*
  - Involvement of multiple organs or systems
  - Brain abnormalities particularly involving the posterior fossa, malformations of cortical development
  - Congenital diaphragmatic hernia (CDH)
  - Bilateral cleft lip and palate (CLAP)
  - Gastrointestinal tract abnormalities—duodenal atresia, tracheoesophageal fistula (TEF), and jejunal atresia
  - Renal conditions such as polycystic/multicystic kidneys
  - Omphalocele

- Skeletal dysplasia
- Radial ray defects
- Cardiac defects—atrioventricular septal defect (AV canal defect—complete/partial), Tetralogy of Fallot, aortic arch anomalies, pulmonary stenosis, and perimembranous VSD (ventricular septal defect)
- Association with early onset fetal growth restriction
- History of consanguinity or previous affected first/second degree relative

Q3. Which defects have less surgery-related mortality and a good quality of life postsurgical correction?

Draft recommendations: Isolated means that the defect should be isolated, chromosomal/genetic associations should be ruled out, and pregnancy should not be complicated by severe prematurity and growth restriction. The defect itself should not be complicating other organ systems.

Following conditions when truly isolated without any associated chromosomal or genetic abnormalities, have a higher cure rate:

- Cleft lip and palate (CLAP)
- Gastroschisis
- Omphalocele
- Lung lesions (without hydrops/pleural effusion)—congenital pulmonary adenomatoid malformations (CPAM), bronchopulmonary sequestration (BPS)
- Abdominal cysts
- Atrial/ventricular septal defect
- Classical Tetralogy of Fallot (TOF)
- Transposition of great arteries
- Truncus arteriosus
- Pulmonary stenosis
- Coarctation of aorta
- Pelviureteric junction (PUJ) obstruction
- Vesicoureteric reflux (VUR)
- Ureterocele
- Anorectal malformation
- Tracheoesophageal fistula (TEF)/esophageal atresia (EA) —outcomes also depend upon the length of esophageal gap
- Duodenal atresia
- Gastrointestinal tract obstruction (length of obstructed segment might affect the long-term outcomes)

Q4. Which defects are at high risk or premature births and in need in-utero transfer to a higher/tertiary care center?

Draft recommendations

The following defects need early referral to a tertiary center:

- All cardiac defects
- Congenital diaphragmatic hernia (CDH)
- Conditions affecting the lung size, e.g., CPAM, BPS, etc.
- Esophageal/duodenal atresia
- Any lesion causing compression on the esophagus or the intestines causing polyhydramnios

Q5. What are the defects in which prognosis depends not only on the defect but the changes caused by it?

Draft recommendations:

- Congenital diaphragmatic hernia—associated lung hypoplasia, and pulmonary hypertension are the main prognostic factors.
- Omphalocele/gastroschisis—bowel ischemia due to constriction at the level of abdominal wall defect can lead to short gut syndrome, the extent of the defect also impacts the outcome.
- Ureterocele/PUJ obstruction/posterior urethral valve—residual renal function guides the prognosis when the back pressure is causing bilateral hydronephrosis. Prenatal prediction of renal function still lacks accuracy.
- Neural tube defects—large defects lead to severe ventriculomegaly that can lead to brain parenchymal damage, a higher level of defect worsens the lower limb mobility and bladder bowel function. Small caudal defects or closed neural tube defects have a better prognosis.
- CPAM/BPS—can lead to hydrops if the lesion is significantly large.

Q6. Is the prognosis different in fetuses with cardiac defects?

Draft recommendations: Prognostication in cardiac defects—it is important to involve a pediatric cardiologist and cardiothoracic vascular surgeon to aid in diagnosing, prognostication, counseling, and managing these cases. Providing social support for delivery and management at tertiary care centers often impacts decision-making.

Summary of evidence: Risk Adjustment for Congenital Heart Surgery for ICD-10 Administrative Data (RACHS-2) is a scoring system that divides surgeries into six categories, Category 1 with the lowest and Category 6 with the highest surgery-related risk. Category 1 surgeries are—ASD repair, VSD repair, coarctation of the aorta without VSD, vascular ring, pacemaker/ICD procedure, pulmonary valve replacement/repair, Konno procedure, aortic stenosis, subvalvular or supravalvular repair, PAPVC repair, aortic valve repair, aortic valve replacement, tricuspid valve repair, aortopexy. Category 2 surgeries—Fontan, Mitral valve repair, PDA closure, surgical, Glenn, arterial switch without VSD, transitional or complete AVC (AVSD) repair, TOF repair with or without ventriculostomy, RV-PA conduit, AP window repair, cardiac tumor resection, pulmonary arterioplasty, anomalous origin of coronary artery from aorta (AOCAA) or from PA (ALCAPA/ARCAPA), cor triatriatum repair, pericardial drainage procedure, pericardiectomy, ventricular aneurysm repair, ASD repair with patch + pulmonary valve replacement, pulmonary valve excision, VSD repair + pulmonary valve replacement, VSD repair + PAPVC repair.

BIBLIOGRAPHY

1. Allen P, Zafar F, Mi J, et al. Risk Stratification for Congenital Heart Surgery for ICD-10 Administrative Data (RACHS-2). J Am Coll Cardiol. 2022;79(5):465-78.
2. Baschat AA, Desiraju S, Bernier ML, et al. Management advances for congenital diaphragmatic hernia: integrating prenatal and postnatal perspectives. Transl Pediatr. 2024;13(4):643-62.
3. Carlsson T, Starke V, Mattsson E. The emotional process from diagnosis to birth following a prenatal diagnosis of fetal anomaly: a qualitative study of messages in online discussion boards. Midwifery. 2017;48:53-9.
4. Chih WL, Tung YH, Lussier EC, et al. Associated factors with parental pregnancy decision-making and use of consultation after a prenatal congenital heart disease diagnosis. Pediatr Neonatol. 2023;64(4):371-80.
5. Fry J, Antiel RM, Michelson K, et al. Ethics in prenatal consultation for surgically correctable anomalies and fetal intervention. Semin Pediatr Surg. 2021;30(5):151102.
6. Gowda M, Thiagarajan M, Satheesh S, et al. Prenatal grading of fetal congenital heart disease and its influence on decision making during pregnancy and postnatal period: a prospective study. J Matern Fetal Neonatal Med. 2022;35(16):3158-66.
7. Lakhoo K. Fetal counselling for surgical conditions. Early Hum Dev. 2012;88(1):9-13.
8. Narang A, Carlsen V, Long A, et al. Anterior abdominal wall defects managed at a tertiary maternal-fetal medicine service in New Zealand: What counselling advice can we offer parents?. Aust N Z J Obstet Gynaecol. 2019;59(6):805-10.
9. Ozyuncu O, Canpolat FE, Ciftci AO, et al. Perinatal outcomes of fetal abdominal cysts and comparison of prenatal and postnatal diagnoses. Fetal Diagn Ther. 2010;28(3):153-59.
10. Rieder W, Maurer SV, Giannoni E, et al. Fetal Omphalocele: Review of Predictive Factors Important for Antenatal Counseling? Obstet Gynecol Surv. 2022;77(11):683-95.
11. Ronai C, Kim A, Dukhovny S, et al. Prenatal Congenital Heart Disease-It Takes a Multidisciplinary Village. Pediatr Cardiol. 2023;44(5):1050-6.

CHAPTER 10

Fetal Surveillance of a "Small Baby"

Prathima Radhakrishnan

INTRODUCTION

KEY QUESTIONS

1. How to differentiate between "fetal size" and "fetal growth"?
2. What is the best way to assess fetal growth and which charts should be used?
3. What are the risk factors for a "small baby" in pregnancy?
4. What is the optimum surveillance pathway for women according to their risk for having a "small baby"?
5. How and why to differentiate an "SGA baby" from a "growth restricted" baby, i.e., FGR?
6. How to differentiate early FGR versus late FGR?
7. What investigations and interventions should be considered when a fetal growth disorder has been diagnosed in the pregnancy?
8. How can the risk of fetal growth disorders in pregnancy be reduced?

Fetal growth is a dynamic process and hence a continuum.

Common definitions used by consensus of experts and national guidelines **(Table 1)**.

Q1. How to differentiate between "fetal size" and "fetal growth"?

Draft recommendations:

- "Fetal size" refers to the biometric measurements, i.e., head circumference (HC), biparietal diameter (BPD), abdominal circumference (AC), femur length (FL), all of which are computed into specific formulae to calculate the estimated fetal weight (EFW).

TABLE 1: International consensus on terminology to be used.

Terminology	*Definition*
Appropriate for gestational age (AGA)	Fetal size between 10th and 90th centile
Small for gestational age (SGA)	Fetal size <10th centile
Fetal growth restriction (FGR)	Fetal size or abdominal circumference (AC) <3rd centile OR if <10th centile with Doppler abnormalities
Static growth	No forward growth velocity in estimated fetal weight (EFW) or AC, at least 14 days apart

- "Fetal growth" is a dynamic process and assessment requires multiple observations of fetal size over time. There should be a minimum of two assessments to define "fetal growth."
- All measurements must be plotted on specific growth chart to determine the trajectory, i.e., growth velocity of the fetus.

Summary of evidence: A single point assessment of fetal biometry, i.e., BPD, HC, AC, and FL will provide information of the fetal size at that point of time. However, to assess the fetal growth which is a function of the change in fetal size over time, the measurements need to be plotted on a growth curve. All fetuses maintain a growth velocity and the potential to achieve this defines "normal growth velocity." Any failure to achieve this refers to "slowing down of the growth" and hence fetal growth restriction.

The two biometric measurements used to compare the growth velocity must be at least 2–3 weeks apart to minimize the false positive rates for detecting FGR/SGA.

Fetal size must be assessed using the HC, AC, and FL by the Hadlock formula which is most accurate and most widely used. The addition of BPD to the formulae does not increase the accuracy as there are considerable variations in the ranges across populations. Hadlock equation estimates fetal size more accurately as compared to the INTERGROWTH-21st equation.

Q2. What is the best way to assess fetal growth and which charts should be used?

Draft recommendations:

- Ultrasound is the core component of fetal growth assessment and surveillance.
- Diagnosis of a fetal growth disorder should be based on high-quality measurements taken by trained personnel.
- Standard views of the BPD, HC, AC, and FL must be obtained as per the reference growth charts that is being used by the personnel.
- Regular audit of the images is recommended to maintain high standard of practice.
- Use of growth charts is essential to assess fetal growth trajectory.
- Current biometry is compared to the previous measurements taken at the anomaly scan to assess the growth velocity.
- The choice of the fetal growth chart must be based on assessment of EFW and not newborn birth weight.

Summary of evidence: Growth scans must be performed by professionally trained personnel as per the recommended standard planes by international guidelines provided by several professional bodies such as the FMF, ISUOG, BMUS, SoR, etc. Quality control of the images and measurements must be a part of ongoing audit. The formula to calculate the EFW must not be changed at subsequent scans as this will impact the diagnosis of a small baby. The method used for measurements must match the method described in the chart that is being used to interpret the growth rate.

There are several fetal growth charts based on population studies, customized based on maternal characteristics, ethnicity, etc. The objective should be to evaluate the individual fetal growth trajectory and deviation, if any, to define a small baby. Hence, when choosing the growth chart, the gestational age, local clinical guidelines, and the population that is being studies must be considered. The most used fetal growth charts are WHO growth standards, INTERGROWTH-21st, charts based on Hadlock formula, customized growth charts (GROW), country and ethnicity specific charts.

A consultation with a fetal medicine specialist consultation would be beneficial to decide the most appropriate growth chart and specific clinical issue.

Evidence gap:

- Audit of images taken for fetal biometry in each unit and comparison between units to maintain standardization especially when there is a migrating pregnant population.
- Evaluate the impact and compare the reference growth charts used in the local population to predict adverse perinatal outcome.
- Determine the action threshold based on the charts as per the local population demographics.
- Adjusting the reference charts as per the local population datasets.

Q3. What are the risk factors for a "small baby" in pregnancy?

Draft recommendations

- Antenatal care must include risk assessment for having a "small baby" and this should be a dynamic process throughout the pregnancy.
- Risk assessment starts at the time of booking with a detailed history, including review of previous obstetric and medical history, examination of the mother, maternal weight and height, current pregnancy parameters, presence of multiple fetuses, ultrasound, and serum markers **(Table 2)**.
- Risk assessment models have been developed by the fetal medicine foundation (FMF) that helps to predict the possibility of developing FGR in the first trimester.
- The "high risk" women identified by the first trimester screening can benefit from prophylactic aspirin, to reduce the effect of placenta dysfunction.
- Other nonpreeclampsia causes of FGR must also be considered as these may be more difficult to predict.

TABLE 2: Level of risk based on clinical findings.

	Factor	*Level of risk*
Maternal charecteristics	Maternal age >40 years	Moderate
	Maternal BMI <18/>35	Moderate
	Maternal weight	Moderate
	Smoking	Moderate
	Drug use/abuse	Moderate
	Ethnicity	Moderate
	Social deprivation	Moderate
	Unmarried status	Moderate
Medical history	Pre-existing medical disorders	High
	Bariatic surgery	High
	Congenital uterine anomalies	Moderate
Obstetric history	Small baby/FGR/preterm birth	High
	Stillbirth	High
	Pregnancy loss	High
	Placenta medicated complications	High
	Short (<6 months)/long (>60 months) interpregnancy interval	Moderate
Antenatal risk factors	Maternal alcohol consumption	Moderate
	Caffeine consumption >300 mg/day	Moderate
	IVF and ICSI	Moderate
Paternal factors	Changing paternity	Moderate
Current pregnancy	Multiple pregnancy	High
Biochemical markers	Low PAPP-A <0.5 MoM	High
	High AFP >2 MoM	High
	High Inhibin >2 MoM	High
Ultrasound markers	Uterine artery Doppler	High
	Echogenic bowel	High
	Single umbilical artery	High
	Fetal biometry 10th centile	High
Developing factors	Maternal diabetes	High
	Maternal hypertension	High
	Bleeding in pregnancy	High
	Maternal infection	High

Source: Adapted from RCOG GTG No. 31.

- In the mid trimester, women may be:
  - "Low risk"—absence of any risk factors, normal anomaly scan and fetal biometry >10th centile—routine antenatal follow-up with measurement of symphysis fundal height (SFM).
  - "Moderate risk"—moderate risk factors, normal anomaly scan and fetal biometry >10th centile—serial SFH measurements and serial ultrasound scan from 30–32 weeks, every 4 weeks.
  - "High risk"—high risk factors; consider prescribing aspirin 150 mg at night if <16 weeks.
    - Assess uterine artery Doppler (UAD) at anatomy scan.
    - Normal UAD + EFW ≥10th centile—serial USS from 32 weeks; every 2–3 weeks till delivery.
    - Normal UAD + EFW <10th centile—serial USS from 26 weeks; every 2–3 weeks till delivery.
    - Abnormal UAD + EFW ≥10th centile—serial USS from 28 weeks; every 2–3 weeks till delivery.
    - Abnormal UAD + EFW <10th centile—discussion with a fetal medicine specialist.
- Women unsuitable for monitoring of fetal growth by measurement of SFH, e.g., BMI >35 kg/m^2, presence of multiple fibroids, etc., must have serial USS from 28–30 weeks every 3–4 weeks.
- If at any point of care, the mother develops any medical complications such as diabetes, hypertension, or bleeding, then serial scans should be performed from diagnosis till delivery.

Summary of evidence: Assessment of risk for having a small baby must be an essential part of antenatal care and is a dynamic process which needs to re-evaluated at every visit. This should be based on previous medical and obstetric history, current demographics, test results (ultrasound and blood tests), and review of previous medical records.

Data from ASPRE and SPREE studies that were primarily conducted for prediction of preeclampsia showed that a high proportion of preterm SGA can be identified and prevented by prophylactic use of aspirin 150 mg nocte till 36 weeks. However, screening for SGA attributed to other causes may need more structured and consistent approach throughout the pregnancy to assess the "level" of risk as this can change with development of new maternal signs and symptoms.

Biochemical markers used for aneuploidy screening in the first trimester, particularly a low PAPP-A is an independent risk factor. Low levels of PAPP-A are known to be associated with stillbirths related to placental dysfunction, abruption, and FGR.

Morris et al. demonstrated that low PAPP-A is associated with SGA below 10th centile (OR 2.08, 95% CI 1.8–2.29), SGA below 5th centile (OR 2.83, 95%

CI 2.52–3.18). In addition, α-fetoprotein (AFP) and inhibin A above 2 MoM are also associated with SGA/FGR. The evidence for low estriol and high beta hCG (>4 MoM) is not reliable though this can be frequently seen with abnormal levels of other second trimester serum screening hormones. The meta-analysis, however, did not support the use of these hormones in isolation as primary screening tools for SGA/FGR. There is no evidence currently for the use of prophylactic aspirin in these women who have abnormal levels of these hormones in the mid trimester.

Fetal biometry below the 10th centile even with normal UAD should prompt for an early reassessment of fetal growth. The FASP guidance suggests that when the measurements are below the 5th centile, the mother should be referred to as fetal medicine specialist to assess for presence of any additional anomalies or markers.

The RCOG guidelines on antenatal care suggests that following antepartum hemorrhage, women should be classified as "high risk" and recommended serial growth scans. Women with chronic hypertension, severe gestational hypertension (BP ≥160/110 mm Hg) and preeclampsia are recommended to have serial assessment of fetal growth by ultrasound as per the NICE guidelines.

Evidence gap:

- Development of prediction model for risk assessment including preexisting and developing risk factors that can be factored into algorithmic approach to make personalized care for the "small fetus." This mostly nullifies the interdependency of risk factors.
- Prediction models for preeclampsia that also predict SGA and FGR, are available on the FMF website. Local adoption, assessment, and maintenance of quality, and finally adaptation to the local population needs ongoing research and audit practices in be put in place.

Q4. What is the optimum surveillance pathway for women according to their risk for having a "small baby"?

Draft recommendations:

- Risk of developing early/late FGR is linked to concurrent risk factors.
- Prevalence of FGR in a population depends upon prediction and detection methods applied to that population.
- Follow-up after risk categorization is suggested as in **Table 3**, albeit reassessment and reassignment of risk must be followed at every visit to improve the detection rate and minimize the false negatives.
- Ultrasound is the cornerstone for diagnosis and surveillance of a "small baby." Hence, training of the personnel performing scans to ensure high quality measurements are obtained and remain consistent, is important.

TABLE 3: Action plan following detection of risk factor.

Risk level	***Parameters based on***	***Action***
Low risk	Clinical examination	
	SFH <10th centile/suboptimal growth	Refer for USS
Moderate risk	Serial assessment of fetal growth at 32 weeks	Scan interval—3–4 weekly
	Fetal growth charts with sonographic estimation of EFW	
High risk	FT screening for SGA as per FMF algorithm	Serial scans from 24 weeks
Monitored in an expert fetal medicine unit	UAD-PI >95% at mid trimester anomaly scan	Serial growth surveillance
	Fetal biometry <10th centile	Serial growth surveillance
	Fetal AC/EFW <3rd centile	Serial scans from 24 weeks
	Suboptimal/static fetal growth	Serial growth surveillance

Source: Adapted from RCOG GTG No. 31.

- When the maternal BMI is >35 vkg/m^2, fetal presentation is unstable, uterus is known to have multiple fibroids, clinical judgment and SFH measurement is likely to be erratic, and in these situations, ultrasound is indicated.
- Following estimation of the fetal size EFW and other individual biometry must be plotted on appropriate growth charts to assess the velocity.
- Individual fetal growth trajectories can be interpreted to help in assessing if there is suboptimal fetal growth.
- Fetuses measuring below the 3rd centile must have a management plan for further monitoring and delivery considered at the appropriate time.
- Women with an abnormal UAD and fetal biometry >10th centile can have a follow-up growth scan at 32 weeks unless there is development of any clinical symptoms. However, if the fetal biometry is below the 10th centile, then follow-up growth scan must be decided as per individual requirement.
- Scan intervals are every 2–4 weeks and needs to be catered as per the fetal requirements and maternal condition.
- FGR is diagnosed when the growth velocity drops by 50% or more in the EFW or the AC centiles.
- Doppler studies of the UA, MCA, and DV helps to identify FGR from SGA and in further management regarding follow-up and decision to deliver.
- Additional monitoring tools such as fetal movement, cCTG, and maternal assessment for development of preeclampsia must be done.

- UAD in the 3rd trimester can be used to assess the possibility of placental dysfunction causing the fetal growth disorder and can be helpful in predicting adverse outcome in suspected SGA in the third trimester.

Summary of evidence

"Low risk" population: The Cochrane meta-analysis comparing abdominal palpation to measurement of the symphysis fundal height (SFH) did not show the latter to be superior in detection of SGA. The NICE guideline suggested that both, SFH and ultrasound assessment were not adequately sensitive in detection of SGA. However, SFH remains a reasonable choice as ultrasound scans may be more challenging especially in resource-limited setting. "Suboptimal growth velocity" (no increase in the SFH measurements taken 2 weeks apart) or if there is any additional clinical finding, then ultrasound assessment of fetal growth must be done. Customized and INTERGROWTH SFH charts are available online. However, the performance of these charts is limited especially in heterogenous populations.

NICE study in 2020 concluded that routine 3rd trimester ultrasound scan in uncomplicated singleton pregnancy did not influence the perinatal mortality and hence cannot be offered routinely, though other comparative studies showed a detection of 57% with routine scan as compared to 20% when scans were performed prompted by a clinical indication.

GC S et al. systematic review on diagnostic performance of ultrasound scan concluded that fetal AC has a higher sensitivity than EFW for a 10% false positive when conducted near term to detect FGR but not SGA. However, in view of increased maternal anxiety, rate of IOL, and iatrogenic prematurity, NICE committee did not recommend routine USS in this population.

"Moderate risk" population: A diagnosis and subsequent decisions regarding management of fetal growth disorders must be based on high quality assessment by appropriately trained personnel. The BMUS and ISUOG provide detailed guidelines on performing the third trimester scan.

Fetal AC is as predictive for SGA and more for neonatal morbidities as per the POP trial. The 10% margin of error with EFW must be recognized when interpreting results and making management decisions. The EFW is affected by the quality of the biometric ultrasound images and hence the importance of quality control.

Fetal biometry must be plotted on appropriate growth chart to assess the growth velocity. Prescriptive charts like those of WHO, country-specific, and INTERGROWTH-21st presume that al fetuses grow under optimal conditions. Customized growth charts such as GROW, adjust to various ethnicities, maternal height, weight, parity, and fetal gender. One specific chart does not fit all. Hence, local adaptation based on the population studied must be considered.

The EFW on the INTERGROWTH-21st is lower as compared to those on Hadlock, WHO and FMF charts. Hence, INTERGROWTH-21st identified only 4.4% of babies with SGA <10th centile and 20.6% LGA >90th centile.

"High risk" population: The RCOG-GTG 31 recommends that all "high risk" women must have UAD Doppler study along with the anomaly scan at 20–24 weeks. Subsequent normalization of the UAD-PI might occur but the risk for SGA in the newborn remains. Hence, follow-up scans need to continue.

Several biomarkers have been studied and proposed as adjuncts to serial ultrasound to identify fetuses that are at high risk of adverse outcome. A high s-flt1/PlGF ratio is recommended for the diagnosis of preeclampsia and detection of associated SGA/FGR. However, the efficacy of prediction in nonhypertensive women remains to be evaluated.

Evidence gap:

- Benefit of routine third trimester scan, including the most appropriate timing to predict the possibility of SGA and FGR needs to be combined with additional biometry and/or biochemical markers to improve prediction, especially in the "low" and "moderate" risk population.
- Risk factors as per ethnicity and local influencing factors may be variable and needs to be established for various populations.
- The optimal timing for screening for SGA/FGR, time interval between scans and cost effectiveness of a screening program needs to be established.
- The reliability of risk categorization as suggested by RCOG needs to be audited for local populations.

Q5. How and why to differentiate an "SGA baby" from a "growth restricted" baby, i.e., FGR?

Draft recommendations:

- A fetus that is below the 10th centile (EFW/AC) and maintaining its growth potential is an SGA baby. The risk of adverse neonatal outcomes for this fetus is lower. However, this baby needs to be monitored serially with growth and Doppler scan to assess for overlapping growth restriction.
- A fetus that fails to reach its growth potential in comparison to the previous scan is a "growth restricted" baby. This may be due to genetic, environmental, fetal, placental, or maternal factors.
- Some, but not all growth restricted fetuses will be small.
- The likelihood of FGR is higher in a small baby.
- A growth restricted fetus is at higher risk of perinatal mortality and morbidity and hence close surveillance is recommended.
- Uteroplacental and fetal Doppler studies are incorporated into the growth scan to differentiate between SGA and FGR fetuses **(Table 4)**.

TABLE 4: Difference between SGA and FGR fetuses.

SGA	***FGR***
Perinatal and long-term outcomes—normal	Perinatal and long-term outcomes—POOR (stillbirth, neonatal death, neurodevelopmental delay, adult-onset disease)
NO IUFD	Risk of IUFD present
No signs of fetal adaptation	Signs of adaptation + (fetal Doppler)
Cause: Unknown (constitutional)	*Cause:* Placental insufficiency

TABLE 5: Definition of early and late FGR fetuses as per Delphi consensus.

Early FGR ***GA <32 weeks*** ***(in absence of congenital anomalies)***	***Late FGR*** ***GA ≥32 weeks*** ***(in absence of congenital anomalies)***
AC/EFW <3rd centile or UA-AEDF/or AC/EFW <10th centile with either and/or 1. Ut. A-PI >95th centile and/or 2. Um. A-PI >95th centile	AC/EFW <3rd centile or at least 2 out of 3 of following: 1. AC/EFW <10th centile 2. AC/EFW crossing centiles >2 quartiles on growth centile 3. CPR <5th centile or Um. A-PI >95th centile

- Use of biophysical profile (BPP) scoring, and computerized CTG should be used to compliment surveillance further.
- Placental biomarkers, especially ratio of soluble FMS-like tyrosine kinase-1 (sFlt-1) and placental growth factor (PlGF) has been used to rule out preeclampsia in suspicious cases. This may be helpful in differentiating between SGA and FGR also as the latter is frequently seen in women with early onset preeclampsia.
- FGR is further subdivided based on gestational at diagnosis—early onset FGR is detected before 32 weeks and late onset FGR is detected after 32 weeks, in the absence of fetal anomalies and defined as per the Delhi consensus **(Table 5)**.
- The differentiation between early and late onset is important as the prevalence, ultrasound findings, management, associated maternal morbidities, and perinatal outcomes varies between the two.

Summary of evidence: Jason Gardosi et al. study showed that unrecognized FGR/SGA accounts to 50% of stillbirths in nonanomalous fetuses.

The SGA refers to a fetus with an EFW/AC below the 10th centile that is well-maintained at the subsequent growth scans. On the other hand, defining FGR can be challenging as there is a need to determine that fetus' growth potential. Hence, additional parameters such as sequential assessment by ultrasound, Doppler studies of fetal and placental vessels, CTG and biomarkers are used. FGR is further subdivided into early and late onset based on the gestational age at diagnosis as per the Delphi consensus. The Delphi consensus-based definition of FGR is proposed to be used currently in clinical practice and research studies.

Blue et al. demonstrated that AC is comparable to EFW in prediction of SGA and LGA. In the prospective pregnancy outcome prediction (POP) study, the addition of AC growth velocity was the only biometric measurement that identified babies at increased risk of neonatal morbidity.

Reduced fetal growth velocity in the third trimester is associated with increased perinatal risks, and hence, detection is likely to improve the outcomes for these babies. A "reduced growth velocity" has been defined as 50% reduction in the growth velocity between two size estimates, i.e., EFW or AC.

EFW/AC below the 10th/5th and 3rd centiles has been studied and the Delphi consensus-based definition of FGR has been widely accepted for clinical practice and future research studies. An EFW/ AC below the 3rd centile or 50% or more drop in the parameter is defined as FGR. However, if the EFW/AC is <10th centile, then additional Doppler abnormality in the uterine or the umbilical artery must be demonstrated. This is to reduce the unnecessary interventions including iatrogenic preterm delivery that can be associated with false positive diagnosis of FGR.

Doppler studies of the uterine and fetal vessels help in assessment of uteroplacental dysfunction leading to suboptimal fetal growth.

Several placental biomarkers, including proteins like mRNA, have been studied in screening, diagnosis, and therapy of placental disease. Pregnancy-related plasma protein-A (PAPP-A) has been used in the first trimester. The ratio of soluble FMS-like tyrosine kinase-1 (sFlt-1) and placental growth factor (PlGF) has been used to rule out preeclampsia in suspicious cases. This may be helpful in differentiating between SGA and FGR as the latter is frequently seen in women with early onset preeclampsia.

Evidence gap:

- Prospective studies to assess the accuracy of the adoption of the Delphi consensus and ISUOG recommendations for early and late FGR for local populations.
- Monitor the fetuses defined to be below the 3rd centile/growth restricted as per the reference chart to assess the true positives.
- Determine the role of biomarkers to delineate early and late onset FGR and if it plays a role in management and decision regarding delivery at the appropriate time. This may be combined with the ultrasound parameters.

Q6. How to differentiate early versus late FGR?

Early onset FGR (eFGR)—considerations

Draft recommendations:

- The fetus does not grow at the expected rate before 32 weeks gestation.
- eFGR is less common (0.3%) as compared to late FGR.
- eFGR can be caused by:
  - *Placental insufficiency*
  - *Maternal health conditions:* Hypertension, preeclampsia, diabetes, or chronic kidney disease.
  - *Genetic, chromosomal, or structural anomalies in the fetus*
  - *Maternal and fetal infections*: Rubella, CMV, and toxoplasmosis.
  - *Lifestyle factors:* Smoking, alcohol use, or drug abuse during pregnancy.

Diagnosis

- Early detection and appropriate management are crucial for improving outcomes.
- When suspected/diagnosed, these pregnancies should be monitored in collaboration with a tertiary care fetal medicine unit with experienced specialists.
- Diagnosis is by ultrasound scan. Fetal biometry plotted on growth chart shows reduced growth velocity associated with changes in amniotic fluid (usually reduced), uteroplacental Doppler studies, presence of markers or structural anomalies in the fetus or stigmata of fetal infections.
- Invasive testing, i.e., amniocentesis must be considered as there is an increased association with chromosomal and genetic anomalies, even in the absence of structural defects visible on the scan.
- Monitoring should include a multimodality assessment including CTG, UA, MCA, and DV Doppler studies and cCTG where available.
- Follow-up assessment must be scheduled as per the severity and changes in the Doppler studies. ISUOG or Barcelona protocol may be followed **(Flowcharts 1 and 2)**.
- Currently, there is no effective therapy for eFGR. However, timely recognition, effective management of maternal condition may prolong the pregnancy and reduce the incidence and effects of severe preterm delivery.
- Timely use of steroids for fetal lung maturity, magnesium sulfate for neuroprotection, in utero transfer to a tertiary care unit with neonatal ICU facilities, and timely delivery via the safest mode are the key to improve the perinatal outcomes. ISUOG or Barcelona protocol may be followed **(Flowcharts 1 and 2)**.
- Prognosis depends upon the severity and cause of the growth restriction in addition to the gestational age at delivery. There is an increased risk or

Flowchart 1: Stage-based decision algorithm for management of FGR.

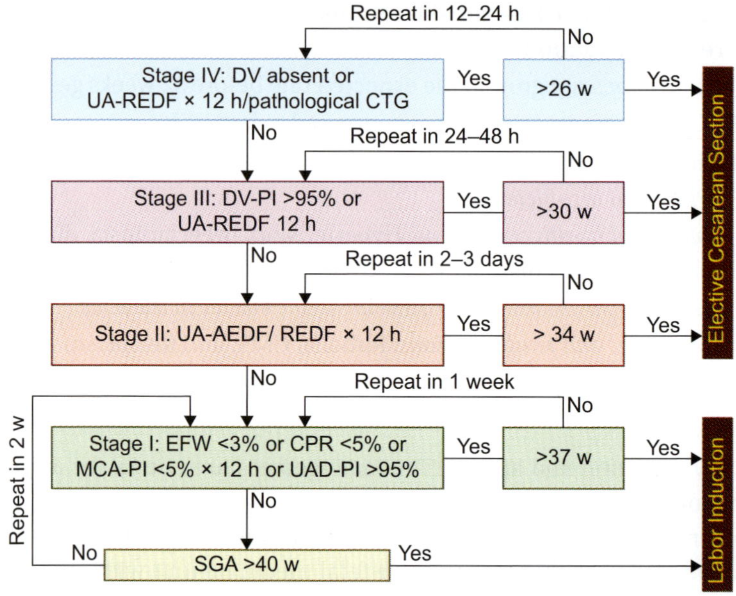

Source: Adapted from uniform management of FGR, Barcelona protocol.

preterm delivery, low birth weight, and developmental issues in short- and long-term for these babies.

- Premature delivery may need to be considered in case of worsening of fetal Doppler/ stress tests or maternal health condition, e.g., worsening of maternal preeclampsia.
- Multidisciplinary management by fetal, maternal and/or other relevant specialists along with appropriate antenatal counseling by neonatal team is recommended.
- There may be a role for biomarkers, especially in the presence of abnormal Doppler studies and maternal preeclampsia.

Summary of evidence: The eFGR is caused by placental dysfunction. Hence, elevated UAD-PI typically precedes the onset of typical changes in other Doppler parameters, fetal heart rate, and BPP changes. The UA, MCA, and DV Doppler show typical patterns and represent cardiovascular and metabolic compromise in the fetus. The rate at which the UA changes from increased PI to absent and then reversal of EDF represents the rate of fetal deterioration. Sometimes, this may be rapid and other times slow, depending upon the severity of the underlying pathology. Further cardiovascular deterioration can lead to reduced STV and repetitive decelerations on the CTG before finally ending in a stillbirth. In addition, studies have shown that, particularly in hypertensive disorders, there is alteration in the placenta mediated

Flowchart 2: Recommended management of pregnancies based on Doppler and cCTG findings.

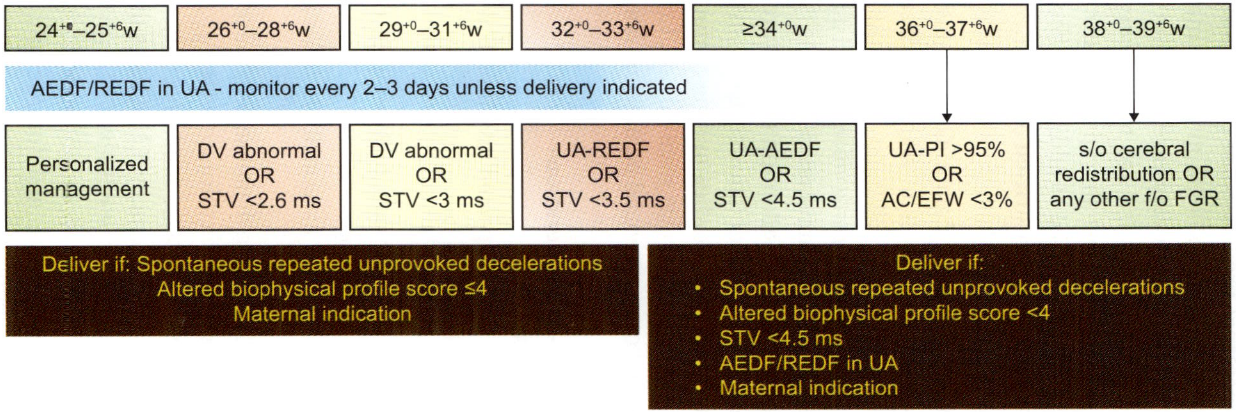

Source: Adapted from ISUOG 2020.

angiogenic factors, i.e., elevation of sFlt-1 and reduction in PlGF leading to an increased ratio, suggestive of worsening placental dysfunction.

There is no effective therapy for eFGR after diagnosis. Early recognition and treatment of maternal preeclampsia can prolong pregnancies to an extent. Timely use of steroids for fetal maturity, magnesium sulfate for neuroprotection, transfer to a tertiary care unit with NICU facilities, and appropriate timing of delivery is the key to improve outcomes for these fetuses. Delivery is only effective therapy. However, the risks of early premature delivery must be weighed as additional effects of prematurity can worsen the outcome for a growth restricted baby.

Evidence gap:

- Follow-up of fetuses deemed to have eFGR/SGA and additional of further ultrasound and serum markers to improve efficacy of prediction of adverse neonatal outcomes.
- Need to define "appropriate growth velocity" and if this applies across all gestational ages and for all parameters.
- Audit at local level following adoption of the Barcelona or the ISUOG protocol for management and decision to deliver in eFGR.
- Placental histopathological studies in fetuses that were confirmed to be FGR antenatally and those that were missed. Comparison of the two will guide as to what otter antenatal parameters may be helpful in better understanding.

Late onset FGR (L-FGR)—considerations

Draft Recommendations

- The fetus fails to grow at the expected rate after 32 weeks of gestation.
- L-FGR can be caused by
  - *Placental insufficiency*
  - *Maternal factors*—hypertension, preeclampsia, or diabetes.
  - *Maternal and fetal infections*
  - *Lifestyle factors*—smoking, malnutrition, or substance abuse during pregnancy.
- This can be more challenging to diagnose because it often presents subtly and may not be evident until the third trimester.
- Diagnosis is by ultrasound scan—fetal biometry is plotted on growth chart shows reduced growth velocity. Changes in the amniotic fluid and Doppler studies, are usually none or subtle.
- These fetuses are at increased risk of sudden intrauterine demise, stillbirth, perinatal morbidity, and long-term neurodevelopmental challenges, especially if undetected or unmanaged.
- Management includes close fetal surveillance with serial growth and Doppler scans followed by timely delivery in a tertiary care center with good NICU facilities.

- Follow-up assessment must be scheduled as per the severity and changes in the Doppler studies. ISUOG or Barcelona protocol may be followed **(Flowcharts 1 and 2)**.
- Steroid and magnesium sulfate may be administered to the mother for fetal maturity and neuroprotection.
- Timing and mode of delivery will depend on the severity and deterioration. ISUOG or Barcelona protocol may be followed **(Flowcharts 1 and 2)**.
- Early delivery may reduce intrauterine demises and stillbirth but might compromise with morbidity associated with prematurity, especially when birth weight is also low.
- Multidisciplinary management by fetal, maternal and/or other relevant specialists along with appropriate antenatal counseling by neonatal team is recommended.

Summary of evidence: The placental changes in L-FGR tend to be milder and nonspecific. Hence, the typical alterations that is seen in eFGR is not seen and neither does it follow the cascade of events. Hence, identification and prediction of these events can be delayed. As the Doppler changes may not be obvious, cerebro-placental ratio (CPR) and umbilical-cerebral ratio (UCR) MCA-PI have been suggested which can identify subtle alterations between the two circulations that may not be appreciated by a single parameter.

The BPP may also become abnormal late and hence may not be so useful to determine monitoring intervals. TRUFFLE study showed that the gestational age at delivery after 32 weeks did not affect the risk of poor neurodevelopmental outcome in these babies. This may be due to reduced tolerance of these fetuses to hypoxia making timely identification even more challenging. Hence, frequent monitoring in these fetuses must be like those with eFGR. Currently, the CPR and MCA-PI is the most important Doppler parameters to monitor L-FGR. When the UA-PI is above the 95th percentile, follow-up Doppler studies must be performed twice/week. A low MCA-PI has been implicated in stillbirth within 5 days. However, the measurement of the MCA-PI can show interobserver variation and hence must be repeated within 24 hours by a specialist to reduce false positives, more so when premature delivery is being planned. BPP score also appears to have a poor predictive value as studies have shown that stillbirths have occurred within a week of a normal BPP score. RCOG recommends corticosteroids prophylaxis up to 36 weeks of pregnancy. Although the DIGITAT study did not consider any Doppler parameter, it showed that a policy of induction of labor (IOL) did not affect the rate of instrumental delivery/cesarean section and adverse neonatal or neurodevelopmental outcome at 2 years of age as compared to a policy of expectant management. However, there were higher number of neonates born with a birth weight below the 3rd centile and mothers with preeclampsia in the expectant management group.

Currently, MCA Doppler must not be used to determine timing of delivery as there is no evidence to support the same. In L-FGR, with only low MCA-PI consideration may be given to induction of labor at 38 completed weeks. However, this is not recommended when the UA Doppler shows absent or reversed EDF. The FHR must be monitored in labor continuously.

Evidence gap:

- Determine the role of MCA Doppler in timing of delivery in L-FGR.
- Comparative studies of CPR and UCR in prediction of adverse neonatal and long-term outcomes in babies born following diagnosis of L-FGR.
- Placental biometry and volume imaging by ultrasound and MRI to assess the functional data may help to delineate the FGR from the non-FGR small babies.
- Improve the ultrasound prediction of EFW by 3D volumetric studies.
- Fractional limb volume has been studied along with fetal biometry to improve the prediction of EFW.

Small for Gestational Age (SGA)—considerations
Draft recommendations:

- A structurally normal fetus that is below the 10th percentile for the EFW/AC and normal Doppler findings is an "SGA" baby.
- This may be associated with accelerated placental aging and hence signs of placental hypoperfusion and altered fetomaternal hemodynamic may be evident on the ultrasound scan and Doppler studies.
- These fetuses are at increased risk of preterm birth and associated perinatal mortality and morbidity, including stillbirth and greater incidence of cesarean section for fetal distress.
- Following diagnosis of an SGA fetus, as the fetal Doppler is usually normal, fortnightly review scans to reassess maintenance of fetal growth and well-being is recommended. ISUOG or Barcelona protocol may be followed **(Flowcharts 1 and 2)**.
- Uterine artery Doppler is helpful in assessing those SGA fetuses that are likely to cross over to become FGR. Hence, when the UAD is above the 95th centile for the GA, surveillance should be more frequent.
- Early SGA or late SGA may progress to FGR and hence Doppler assessment and thorough evaluation for "brain sparing" as measured by the cerebro-placental ratio (CPR) or UCR is recommended.
- In SGA babies, it is reasonable to consider delivery between 38 and 39 weeks to reduce the term stillbirth rate without increasing the prematurity rate. ISUOG or Barcelona protocol may be followed **(Flowcharts 1 and 2)**.
- Induction of labor with continuous fetal heart rate monitoring in labor is beneficial as it helps to reduce the rate of emergency cesarean section and operative vaginal delivery.

- Specialized neonatal care is essential, as these babies are more prone to hypoglycemia due to reduced glycogen stores and temperature instability.
- Long-term follow-up is recommended as developmental issues have been reported in these kids.
- SGA fetuses require careful monitoring and management to ensure the best possible outcomes for both the mother and the baby.

Summary of evidence: An SGA baby is a constitutionally small baby that is otherwise structurally normal and with normal Doppler studies. Customized growth charts may be helpful to reduce the false positives. Despite normal fetoplacental Doppler, there is evidence of accelerated placental aging, placental hypoperfusion, low umbilical vein blood flow, altered maternal hemodynamic, and a higher incidence of cesarean section for fetal distress in the fetuses detected to be SGA. This suggests that these fetuses get adapted to the in-utero environment and hence difficult to identify as being "at risk" by routine methods.

The UAD is assessed at the time of diagnosis of SGA and need not be repeated. Late SGA with UAD-PI above the 95th centile is more likely to cross over to FGR and hence needs to be monitored closely for developing "brain sparing". This can happen with late SGA with normal UAD too, albeit less frequently.

The DIGITAT study showed that IOL at 38–39 weeks with continuous FHR monitoring in labor is better than expectant management, especially in the absence of critical UA Doppler findings. The major cause of perinatal death is term stillbirth in these fetuses.

Evidence gap:

- Identify the subgroup of fetuses that is likely to "cross-over" to become FGR based on additional biometry, screening tests performed in the pregnancy and maternal conditions.
- Audit of fetuses reported to be SGA and that were true and false positives delivered after 37 completed weeks to provide accurate detection rates.
- Neonatal outcomes of the prenatally detected SGA babies born after 37 weeks.
- Comparison of the antenatal EFW with the birth weight to determine the margin of error and explore methods to reduce the margins of error.

Q7. What investigations and interventions should be considered when a fetal growth disorder has been diagnosed in the pregnancy?

Draft recommendations:

- Early referral to a specialized fetal medicine unit must be considered.
- Invasive testing to assess for possibility of chromosomal anomalies, copy number variants, and fetal infections, especially CMV, Rubella, and Zika should be offered, especially eFGR.

- Maternal screening for malaria and syphilis should be considered.
- There are no proven interventions in SGA and FGR other than birth of the baby.
- LMWH should not be prescribed after diagnosis of FGR.
- PDE5 inhibitors, sildenafil have not shown to be beneficial or improve outcomes in FGR babies.
- Induction of labor is not contraindicated in SGA fetuses with normal Doppler.
- Antenatal corticosteroids must be offered to women who are at increased risk of preterm delivery between 24 and 34 weeks. Beyond 35 weeks, the risk and benefits must be balanced.
- Intrauterine transfer to appropriate tertiary care unit must be considered to optimize the outcome for the neonate.
- Magnesium sulfate for neuroprotection must be offered to all women at risk of delivery between 24 and 29 weeks and considered for those delivering between 30 and 34 weeks.
- The incidence of cesarean delivery is increased when there is umbilical artery AEDF. IOL may be considered in near term SGA/FGR babies with positive EDF in the umbilical artery.
- Postdelivery histopathological and genetic examination of the placenta must be suggested to assess the cause for SGA/FGR as this will help to assess the risk of recurrence and manage the subsequent pregnancies.
- Postnatal follow-up and counseling must be offered to all women to discuss the preventive strategies for the future.
- Modifiable risk factors such as lifestyle changes and medical conditions must be addressed and treated optimally.

Summary of evidence: Borrell A et al. in their systematic review showed that chromosomal microarray analysis (CMA) had a 4% and 10% higher yield over karyotyping in the absence and presence of structural anomalies with FGR. Prenatal exome however has limited values so far. Additionally, Trisomies 18 and 21 have been reported with SGA, especially when the femur length (FL) is measured below the 5th centile at the mid trimester anomaly scan. A short FL increases the risk of SGA and PTB by 4-times. The RCOG-GTG 31 recommends offering invasive diagnostic testing to all severe SGA fetuses in the presence of structural anomalies and to be considered even in the absence of anomalies and with normal UAD.

SGA can be due to fetal infections, especially CMV, rubella, malaria, and syphilis, and hence these need to be tested in the mother and if possible, on the amniotic fluid.

The RCOG-GTG 31 and ISUOG do not support the use of any form of medical intervention, i.e., LMWH, sildanafil, or PDE5 inhibitors once the diagnosis of FGR has been made.

A Cochrane review of the small baby at term showed no difference in perinatal or long-term outcome in premature delivery versus expectant management policies.

The RCOG-GTG and ISUOG recommend IOL at 37^{+0} to 38^{+6} weeks in small babies with Doppler changes. However, if only the fetal biometry is below the 10th centile and FGR has been excluded, IOL may be considered at 39 weeks.

The RCOG guidance recommends antenatal corticosteroids and magnesium sulfate for neuroprotection when the risk for preterm delivery is high.

In the presence of abnormal Doppler, elective cesarean delivery may be considered as there is high chance of intrapartum fetal distress, compromise, and emergency cesarean section.

Postdelivery of a small baby, appropriate investigations, including placental histopathological studies, maternal acquired thrombophilia, and genetic consultation must be performed to identify the cause.

Lifestyle changes, modifiable risk factors, and any medical condition should be optimized so that preventive care can be instituted in future pregnancies to reduce the risk of recurrence. Thorough counseling of the couple about the events would be helpful.

Evidence gap:

- Audit of the presence of CNVs and chromosomal anomalies with isolated FGR.
- Histopathological studies of the placenta and postnatal studies in the short and long term of the babies diagnosed and undiagnosed antenatally must be done to compare the benefit of antenatal detection of SGA and effect on the reduction of adverse outcomes.
- Long-term physical and mental effects on the mother of a difficult pregnancy requiring intensive counseling and frequent scans and the effect of adverse perinatal events if any.

Q8. How can the risk of fetal growth disorders in pregnancy be reduced?

Draft recommendations:

- General measures—reduce smoking, alcohol consumption, drug dependency, and promotion of healthy lifestyle.
- Dietary modification—balanced energy and protein supplementation has shown to be associated with a reduction in SGA baby and increase in mean birth weight.
- Vitamin D 10 μg/day and folic acid 400 μg/day should be continued throughout the pregnancy to reduce the risk of preeclampsia.
- Antiplatelet agents—prevention of preeclampsia with aspirin is most effective when started between 11^{+0} and 16^{+6} weeks of pregnancy. A modest reduction in SGA may be achieved when initiated before 16 weeks. A dose of 100–150 mg was most effective and safe.

- SGA/FGR is more likely related to the underlying disease and hence use of antihypertensive drug therapy for hypertension can help to prolong the pregnancy to a certain extent but does not necessarily reduce the risk of SGA/FGR.

Summary of evidence: Ota et al. suggested that a balanced energy/protein supplementation is associated with reduction in SGA (RR 0.79, 95% CI 0.69–0.90) and an increase in mean birth weight (+40.96 g, 95% CI 4.66–77.26) but protein supplementation alone did not benefit.

Dietary supplements, minerals, micronutrients, and vitamins—omega-3 long chain polyunsaturated fatty acids, multiple micronutrient supplementation, high dose folic acid, and calcium or magnesium supplementation have not shown to reduce SGA consistently in large RCTs nor in Cochrane review of trials.

Fogacci et al. suggested that vitamin D supplementation might be useful to reduce preeclampsia. However, other systematic reviews have not shown benefit in reduction of preeclampsia nor SGA/FGR. In the absence of convincing evidence high doses of vitamin supplements for women at increased risk of SGA/FGR is not recommended.

Roberge et al. established that aspirin when started before 16 weeks was associated with a significant reduction in SGA (RR 0.76, 95% CI 0.61–0.94), but not after 16 weeks. A dose of 100–150mgs taken in the evening or night was more effective than in the morning. RCOG guidelines suggest stopping aspirin at 36 weeks, in view of risk of postpartum hemorrhage.

The RCOG GTG does not recommend the use of LMWH to prevent SGA/FGR irrespective of the presence or absence of thrombophilia.

Progesterone and hydroxychloroquine had not shown to be of benefit in reducing SGA/FGR or preeclampsia and hence not recommended outside of research setting.

Antihypertensive drug therapy for hypertension in pregnancy can help to prolong the pregnancy to a certain extent but has not reduce the risk of SGA/FGR that is likely to be related to the underlying condition. The association of beta blockers and SGA is also inconclusive.

Evidence gap:

- Audit of women identified to be at increased risk (>1 in 100) at the first trimester screening at 11^{+0} to 13^{+6} weeks of pregnancy, practice of prescribing appropriate doses of aspirin, patient compliance in taking the correct dose till 36 weeks and finally outcome measures.
- Placental histopathological studies in fetuses that were at "increased risk" of SGA determined antenatally.
- Future pharmacological interventions after the diagnosis of FGR based on various causes to reduce the adverse neonatal outcomes.

BIBLIOGRAPHY

1. Blue NR, Yordan JMP, Holbrook BD, et al. Abdominal circumference alone versus estimated fetal weight after 24 weeks to predict small or large for gestational age at birth: A meta-analysis. Am J Perinatol. 2017;34(11):1115-24.
2. Boers KE, Vijgen SM, Bijlenga D, et al.; DIGITAT study group. Induction versus expectant monitoring for intrauterine growth restriction at term: randomised equivalence trial (DIGITAT). BMJ. 2010;341:c7087.103.
3. Borrell A, Grande M, Pauta M, et al. Chromosomal microarray analysis in fetuses with growth restriction and normal karyotype: A systematic review and meta-analysis. Fetal Diagn Ther. 2018;44(1):1-9.
4. Bricker L, Medley N, Pratt JJ. Routine ultrasound in late pregnancy (after 24 weeks' gestation). Cochrane Database Syst Rev. 2015;(6):CD001451.
5. Fogacci S, Fogacci F, Banach M, et al. Vitamin D supplementation and incident preeclampsia: A systematic review and meta-analysis of randomized clinical trials. Clin Nutr. 2020;39(6):1742-52.
6. Lees CC, Stampalija T, Baschat AA, et al. ISUOG Practice Guidelines: diagnosis and management of small-for-gestational-age fetus and fetal growth restriction. Ultrasound Obstet Gynecol. 2020;56:298-312.
7. Molina LCG, Odibo L, Zientara S, et al. Validation of Delphi procedure consensus criteria for defining fetal growth restriction. Ultrasound Obstet Gynecol. 2020;56(1):61-6.
8. Morris RK, Bilagi A, Devani P, et al. Association of serum PAPP- A levels in first trimester with small for gestational age and adverse pregnancy outcomes: systematic review and meta-analysis. Prenat Diagn Mar. 2017;37(3):253-65.
9. Morris RK, Cnossen JS, Langejans M, et al. Serum screening with Down's syndrome markers to predict pre-eclampsia and small for gestational age: systematic review and meta-analysis. BMC Pregnancy Childbirth. 2008;8:33.
10. National Institute for Health and Care Excellence. (2021). Antenatal care routine third trimester ultrasound for fetal growth. [online] Available from https:// www. nice. org. uk/guidance/ng201/evidence/q-routine-third-trimester-ultrasound-for-fetal-growth-pdf-331305934364 [Last accessed November, 2024].
11. National Institute for Health and Care Excellence. Antenatal care. [online] Available from https://www.nice. org.uk/guidance/ng201/ [Last accessed November, 2024].
12. Ota E, Hori H, Mori R, et al. Antenatal dietary education, and supplementation to increase energy and protein intake. Cochrane Database Syst Rev. 2015;(6):CD000032.
13. Roberge S, Nicolaides K, Demers S, et al. The role of aspirin dose on the prevention of preeclampsia and fetal growth restriction: systematic review and meta-analysis. Am J Obstet Gynecol. 2017;216(2):110-20.e6.
14. Robert Peter J, Ho JJ, Valliapan J, et al. Symphysial fundal height (SFH) measurement in pregnancy for detecting abnormal fetal growth. Cochrane Database Syst Rev. 2015;(9):CD008136.
15. Rodger MA, Gris JC, de Vries JIP, et al. Low-molecular-weight heparin and recurrent placenta-mediated pregnancy complications: a meta-analysis of individual patient data from randomised controlled trials. Lancet. 2016; 388(10060):2629-41.

16. Sovio U, White IR, Dacey A, et al. Screening for fetal growth restriction with universal third trimester ultra sonography in nulliparous women in the Pregnancy Outcome Prediction (POP) study: a prospective cohort study. Lancet. 2015;386(10008):2089-97.
17. StampalijaT, ThorntonJ, MarlowN, et al.; on behalf of the TRUFFLE-2 Group. Fetal cerebral Doppler changes and outcome in late preterm fetal growth restriction: prospective cohort study. Ultrasound Obstet Gynecol. 2020;56: 173-81.
18. Stirnemann J, Villar J, Salomon LJ, et al. for the International Fetal and Newborn Growth Consortium for the 21st Century (INTERGROWTH-21st), Scientific Advisory Committee, Steering Committees, INTERGROWTH-21st, INTERBIO-21st, Executive Committee, In addition for INTERBIO 21st, Project Coordinating Unit, Data Analysis Group, Data Management Group, In addition for INTERBIO 21st, Ultrasound Group, In addition for INTERBIO-21st:, Anthropometry Group, In addition for INTERBIO-21st:, Laboratory Processing Group, Neonatal Group, Environmental Health Group, Neurodevelopment Group, Participating countries and local investigators, In addition for INTERBIO-21st:, In addition for INTERBIO- 21st. International estimated fetal weight standards of the INTERGROWTH- 21. Ultrasound Obstet Gynecol Apr 2017;49(4):478-86.
19. Tan MY, Poon LC, Rolnik DL, et al. Prediction and prevention of small- for-gestational- age neonates: evidence from SPREE and ASPRE. Ultrasound Obstet Gynecol. 2018;52(1):52-9.
20. The British Medical Ultrasound Society. Professional guidance for fetal growth scans performed after 23 weeks of gestation. [online] Available from https://www.bmus.org/policies- statements- guide lines/ profession al- guidance/ guidance- pages/ profession al- guidance- for- fetal- growth- scans- performed- after- 23- weeks-of-gestation/ [Last accessed November, 2024].

CHAPTER 11

USG and Biochemical Screening in Pregnancy: Key Questions, Recommendations, and Evidence Review

Narendra Malhotra, Jaideep Malhotra, Neharika Malhotra

Q1. What is the primary goal of USG and biochemical screening in pregnancy?

Importance of USG and biochemical bcreening:

- *Purpose:* The goal of both USG and biochemical screening is to identify pregnancies at risk for chromosomal anomalies, structural defects, and other fetal conditions early on, ensuring timely intervention.
- *Benefit to parents:* These screenings provide reassurance to expectant parents, allow for early diagnosis of conditions, and offer the chance to make informed decisions regarding the pregnancy.

Draft recommendations:

- Early identification of fetal structural abnormalities.
- Assessment of chromosomal abnormalities, such as Down syndrome, Edward syndrome, Patau syndrome, and others.
- Screening for maternal conditions like placental insufficiency (by use of color Doppler).
- Facilitate informed decision-making regarding pregnancy continuation or intervention.

Summary of evidence:

- USG identifies fetal structural anomalies with high sensitivity, especially in the second trimester (18–22 weeks). Biochemical screening enhances detection of chromosomal abnormalities.
- First-trimester USG combined with biochemical markers improves early detection of trisomy 21.
- *Evidence supports integrated screening (USG + biochemical markers) (eFTS:* extended first trimester screening as more accurate than either modality alone (Smith et al., 2022).
- NIPS/NIPT is emerging as a very accurate screening tool in current status.

Research gap: Limited data on the integration of new technologies like *artificial intelligence (AI)* in ultrasound interpretation.

Q2. When should USG and biochemical screening be conducted during pregnancy?

Ultrasound screening:

Overview: Ultrasound (USG) is a crucial imaging modality used at various stages of pregnancy to evaluate fetal growth, placental location, amniotic fluid levels, and to detect structural anomalies.

Timing and types

- *First-trimester ultrasound (11–14 weeks):*
    - This scan is combined with biochemical markers (such as PAPP-A and beta-hCG) to assess the risk for trisomy 21 (Down syndrome), trisomy 18, and trisomy 13.
    - The nuchal translucency (NT) measurement is key to identifying chromosomal abnormalities.
    - First trimester fetal anomaly scan by high resolution TVS and 3D–4D ultrasound.
    - Color Doppler in first trimester for preeclampsia prediction and fetal cardiac evaluation.
- *Second-trimester ultrasound (18–22 weeks):*
    - Also known as the anomaly scan, it assesses fetal anatomy in detail and can detect major structural abnormalities such as neural tube defects, congenital heart defects, and skeletal malformations.
    - Plotting of growth charts for identification of fetal growth abnormalities.
    - Use of color Doppler for fetal placental function and early growth restriction.
- *Third-trimester ultrasound (after 28 weeks):* Focuses on fetal growth, position, amniotic fluid levels, and placental location. Doppler studies assess blood flow and help identify issues like fetal growth restriction (FGR).

Interpretation:

- *Normal findings:* Indicate a low likelihood of structural and fetal growth anomalies.
- *Abnormal findings:* Require further investigation, often involving more detailed imaging or additional screening tests.

Biochemical screening:

Overview: Biochemical screening involves testing maternal blood for specific markers that, when combined with USG findings, can indicate the risk of chromosomal abnormalities. These markers include pregnancy-associated plasma protein A (PAPP-A), human chorionic gonadotropin (β-hCG), and others depending on the trimester.

Types

- *First-trimester screening (11–14 weeks):*
  - Involves measuring PAPP-A and free β-hCG (dual marker test).
  - These markers, combined with nuchal translucency from USG, estimate the risk for Down syndrome and other chromosomal disorders (combined screening tests).
  - Penta marker in first trimester and eFTS.
- *Second-trimester screening (15–22 weeks):*
  - Also known as the quadruple test, it measures α-fetoprotein (AFP), hCG, estriol, and inhibin A.
  - Elevated AFP levels may indicate neural tube defects, while abnormal levels of the other markers suggest trisomies 21 and 18.

Interpretation:

- *Low risk:* Suggests a lower likelihood of chromosomal or structural abnormalities.
- *High risk:* Indicates the need for further diagnostic tests, such as chorionic villus sampling (CVS) or amniocentesis.

Draft recommendations:

- First-trimester USG between 11 and 13 weeks 6 days for nuchal translucency measurement and other markers.
- First-trimester biochemical screening between 11 and 14 weeks (extended FTS, Dual marker only, Penta Marker, eFTS, NIPS).
- Second-trimester USG anomaly scan between 18 and 22 weeks.
- Second-trimester biochemical screening between 15 and 22 weeks (Quadruple marker and NIPS).

Summary of evidence:

- Studies show that the 11–14 week window for combined first trimester USG and biochemical screening optimally detects chromosomal abnormalities (Norton et al., 2019).
- Second-trimester USG is considered gold standard for identifying structural abnormalities (Nicolaides et al., 2020).

Research gap: Insufficient evidence on the benefit of *routine third-trimester USG* in low-risk pregnancies, beyond growth monitoring.

Q3. What specific biochemical markers are used in pregnancy screening (Table 1A and B)?

Aneuploidy and preeclampsia testing. (A) Aneuploidy screening in first trimester; (B) Preeclampsia screening in first trimester.

TABLE 1A: Aneuploidy screening in first trimester.

First trimester markers		***DR%***	***FPR%***
PAPP-A + free hCGβ +	PIGF +AFP	80%	5%
PAPP-A + free hCGβ +	PIGF +AFP +NT	90%	1.4%

Modeled performance: Suresh et al, 2017: Submitted for publication.

TABLE 1B: Preeclampsia screening in first trimester.

	PE <32 weeks	***PE <37 weeks***
Maternal history with:	***DR %***	***DR %***
PIGF + PAPP-A	88%	66%
PIGF + PAPP-A + uPTI + MAP	100%	80%

Draft recommendations

- PAPP-A and β-hCG in the first trimester for trisomy risk assessment.
- AFP, hCG, estriol, and inhibin-A in the first and second-trimester quadruple test or Penta Marker test **(Tables 2 and 3)**.
- Noninvasive prenatal testing (NIPT) for fetal DNA analysis.
- Monitor additional emerging biomarkers for more comprehensive screening.

Summary of evidence:

- PAPP-A and β-hCG combined with nuchal translucency measurement in first trimester provide over 85% sensitivity for detecting trisomy 21 (Wald et al., 2018).
- The *quadruple test* in the second trimester improves detection rates for Down syndrome and neural tube defects (Spencer et al., 2021).
- NIPT gives 98–99% accuracy for aneuploidies at 13, 18, and 21.

Research gap: Emerging biochemical markers and *proteomics* are under-researched in routine clinical practice.

Q4. How effective is the combination of USG and biochemical screening in detecting Down syndrome?

Integration of USG and Biochemical Screening (Flowchart 1):

- Sequential screening: Combines first-trimester biochemical markers and nuchal translucency with second-trimester ultrasound and biochemical markers for a more comprehensive risk assessment **(Table 1 A and B)**.
- Contingent screening: Uses first-trimester screening results to determine whether second-trimester testing is necessary **(Table 2)**.
- *Noninvasive prenatal testing (NIPT):* More advanced biochemical screening that uses fetal DNA in the maternal bloodstream to screen for chromosomal abnormalities, offering higher accuracy.

TABLE 2: Comparison of double marker and penta screening.

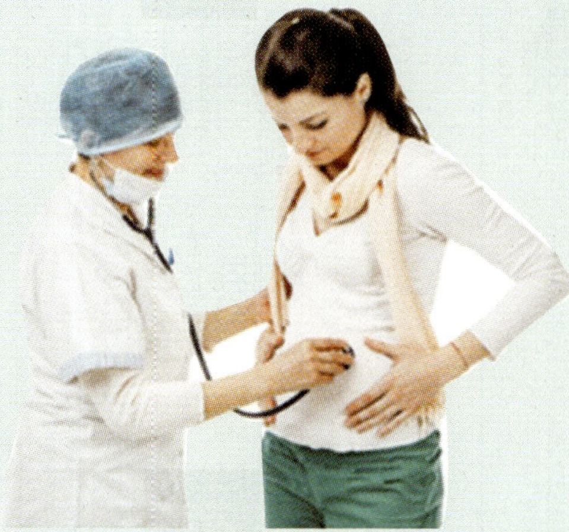

A pentastic journey toward motherhood. First trimester pregnancy/Penta marker screening.

Parameters	Double marker screening	Penta marker screening
Markers analyzed	PAPP-A and free β hCG	PAPP-A, free β hCG, AFP, PIGF, DIA
Detection rate (DR) and false positive rate (FPR) using serum	• At 1/300 cutoff risk the DR of Down syndrome is 86% at 8.4% FPR • At 1/150 cut off risk, the DR of Edward syndrome is 80% at 3.3% FPR and the DR of Patau syndrome is 60% at 0.5% FPR	• At 1/300 cut off risk the DR of Down Syndrome is 92% at 4.8% FPR • At 1/150 cutoff risk, the DR of Edward and Patau syndrome is 88% at 1.2% FPR
Need for further investigation	Requires increased number of follow-on testing, leading to higher costs and anxiety to parents	Reduces the need for follow-on testing by >50%
Preeclampsia detection (A high risk condition during pregnancy that leads to high blood pressure, elevated protein levels, kidney damage, and preterm delivery)	Not detected	Detected

TABLE 3: First trimester screening.

B	Blood pressure	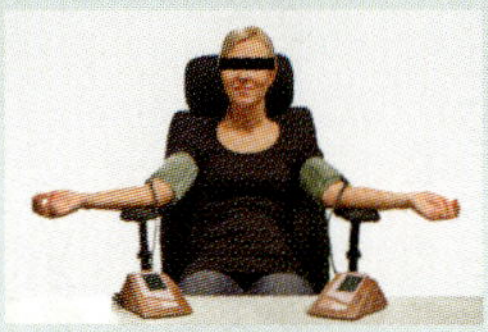 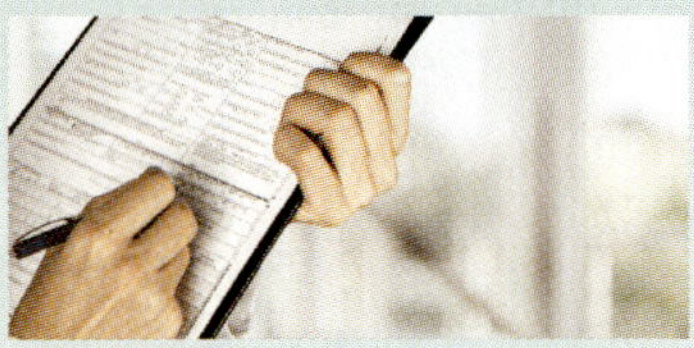
E	Extended clinical history	
H	hCGB	*Turn-around time:* 3 days from the receipt of sample *Results reported:* • *Elevated AFP:* Indicate high risks for structural fetal anomalies and placental problems in pregnancy • *High-risk pre-term PE:* Prophyolaxis with Aspirin 150 mg at bedtime • *High-risk aneuploidy:* Early prenatal diagnosis using classical cytogenetics or prenatal/karyolite BoBs or genetic testing through DNA sequencing *How to order:* Ask a PerkinElmer representative to provide enrolment form along with test requisition form and sample collection kit
A	α-fetoprotein	
P	PAPP-A	
P	PLGF	
Y	Your first trimester scan	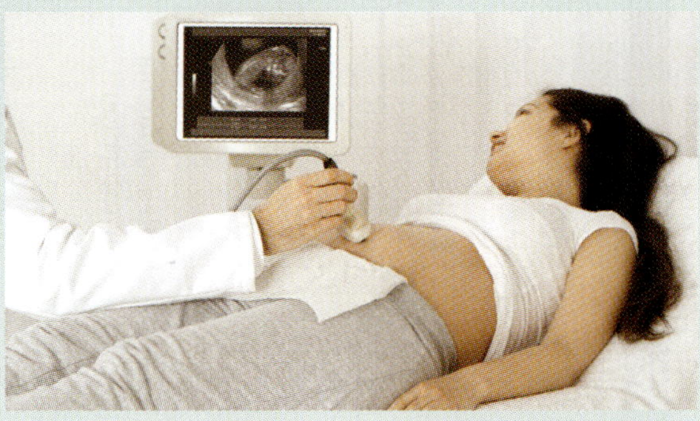

Flowchart 1: New screening protocol.

New screening protocol for trisomy 21 + PE + ONTDs in indian scenario

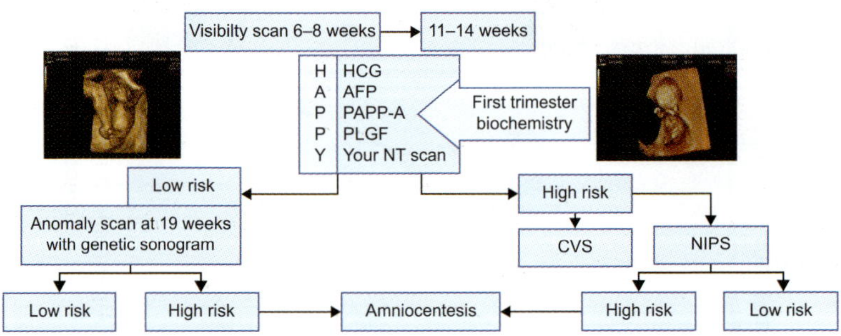

Draft recommendations:

- Combine first-trimester USG (nuchal translucency) with biochemical screening for highest sensitivity. eFTP (Penta marker and be Happy tests improve the accuracy).
- Use *NIPS/NIPT* for women with high-risk results from initial screening or NIPS/NIPT can also be used as primary screening test.
- Follow up abnormal screening results with diagnostic testing (amniocentesis or CVS).
- Regularly update screening protocols to include new evidence-based tools.

Summary of evidence:

- Studies show *combined first-trimester screening* has over 90% detection rate for Down syndrome, particularly when USG and biochemical markers are used together (Gil et al., 2020).
- NIPT has 99% sensitivity and 99% specificity in detecting trisomy 21 (Palomaki et al., 2019).

Research gap: A lack of long-term cost-benefit analysis for implementing *NIPS/NIPT* universally.

Q5. How reliable are second-trimester USG and biochemical markers in detecting neural tube defects (NTDs)?

Role in Detecting Fetal Anomalies:

- *Down syndrome:* Both USG and biochemical markers (low PAPP-A and high β-hCG) are useful for early detection.
- *Neural tube defects:* Elevated AFP in biochemical screening and detailed second-trimester ultrasound can detect conditions like spina bifida.
- *Cardiac and skeletal abnormalities:* Ultrasound in the second trimester is critical for identifying heart defects and skeletal dysplasia.
- *Other chromosomal abnormalities:* USG markers such as nasal bone absence, echogenic bowel, and biochemical markers help in identifying trisomy 21, 18, and 13.

Draft recommendations:

- Perform *second-trimester USG* between 18 and 22 weeks for NTDs and other fetal anomalies.
- Use *AFP levels* from the second-trimester screening for NTD risk assessment.
- Consider genetic counseling if elevated AFP is detected.
- Investigate additional biochemical markers for higher sensitivity.

Summary of evidence:

- *AFP* remains the gold standard biomarker for NTDs, with sensitivity of over 75% (Moore et al., 2021).

- Second-trimester USG has high accuracy in identifying spina bifida and other NTDs (Morris et al., 2020).

Research gap: The addition of *other biochemical markers* for earlier detection of NTDs needs further exploration.

Q6. How does Noninvasive Prenatal Screening/Testing (NIPS) (NIPT) compare to traditional biochemical screening?

Draft recommendations

- Offer NIPS/NIPT as a secondary test for women at high risk for chromosomal abnormalities.
- Expand NIPS/NIPT accessibility for low-risk pregnancies with counseling on limitations.
- Combine NIPS/NIPT with early USG for comprehensive screening.
- Educate healthcare providers on the sensitivity and limitations of NIPS/NIPT.

Summary of evidence

- NIPT/NIPS is highly effective with over 99% accuracy in detecting common trisomies like Down syndrome and Edward syndrome (Bianchi et al., 2019).
- Traditional biochemical screening combined with USG still offers high detection rates but lacks NIPTs precision.
- Extended NIPS/NIPT tests are now available to detect chromosomal microdeletions and twenty two chromosomes.

Research gap: Limited data on the long-term psychological impact of *false positives* in NIPS/NIPT.

Q7. What are the potential risks and limitations associated with USG and biochemical screening?

Limitations of screening:

- *False positives/negatives:* Both USG and biochemical screening can sometimes give misleading results, leading to unnecessary anxiety or false reassurance.
- *Not diagnostic:* These screenings only indicate the likelihood of a condition and do not confirm a diagnosis, requiring invasive testing (like amniocentesis) for definitive diagnosis.

Draft recommendations:

- Ensure that USG is performed by trained professionals to avoid false positives or negatives.
- Avoid unnecessary invasive tests based solely on biochemical screening and age related a priori risk.

- Offer genetic counseling for high-risk pregnancies to interpret results accurately.
- Research on the safety of newer biomarkers and USG techniques should be prioritized.

Summary of evidence:

- USG is generally safe, but *false positives* can lead to unnecessary stress and invasive tests like amniocentesis, which carry a 1% risk of miscarriage (Tabor et al., 2018).
- Biochemical screening has a small risk of *false positives,* which can lead to unnecessary further testing (Gil et al., 2020).
- NIPS is almost 99% accurate for trisomy 13, 18, and 21 and 90% for sex chromosome anomalies.

Research gap: Insufficient research on *long-term effects* of repeated USG exposure. Till date no side effects of ultrasound, in pregnancy to fetus, have been seen.

Q8. How are results of USG and biochemical screening interpreted?

Draft recommendations:

- Use a risk algorithm combining USG and biochemical results **(Flowchart 2)**.
- Incorporate patient age and medical history into screening algorithms.
- Offer further diagnostic testing for pregnancies flagged as high-risk.
- Utilize specialist consultations for abnormal results.

Summary of evidence:

- *Combined risk algorithms* including maternal age, USG, and biochemical results yield higher accuracy for aneuploidy detection (Wald et al., 2018).
- Studies highlight the importance of clinician expertise in interpreting complex screening results (Nicolaides et al., 2020).
- FOSGI TOG (2018–2019) suggested screening protocol **(Table 1)**.

Research gap: Lack of *standardized interpretation protocols* across various healthcare systems.

Q9. What are the socioeconomic impacts of widespread USG and biochemical screening?

Draft recommendations:

- Implement universal access to first-trimester USG and biochemical screening for all pregnant women
- Develop subsidized programs for low-income populations.
- Offer education on the benefits and limitations of screening.
- Assess the cost-effectiveness of NIPS/NIPT in low- and middle-income countries.

Flowchart 2: Genetic screening protocol.

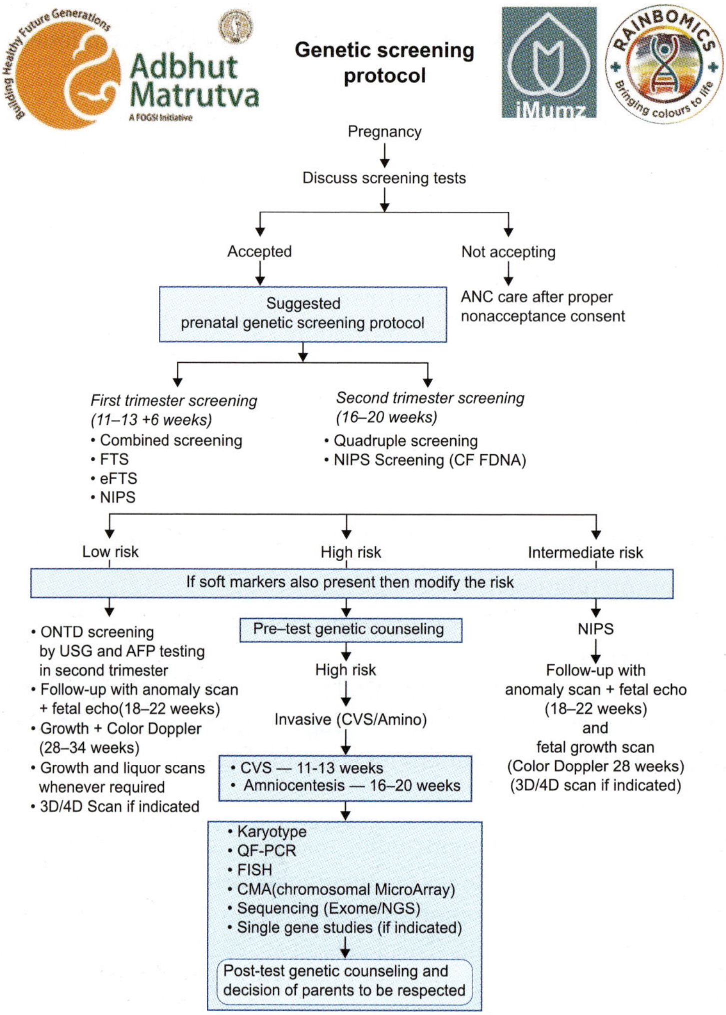

Summary of evidence:

- Evidence shows that *universal access* to USG and biochemical screening improves prenatal care outcomes (Bianchi et al., 2019).
- Socioeconomic disparities remain a barrier to widespread screening, particularly with the high cost of NIPS (Palomaki et al., 2019).

Research gap: A need for studies on the *long-term socioeconomic benefits* of routine screening programs.

Q10. What future developments could enhance USG and biochemical screening in pregnancy?

Draft recommendations

- Invest in *AI and machine learning* for improving USG diagnostic accuracy.
- Expand research into *proteomics* and novel biochemical markers.
- Develop more affordable and accessible versions of NIPT/NIPS.
- Explore advanced imaging techniques for earlier detection of fetal abnormalities.

Summary of evidence:

- Studies are emerging on the use of *AI-assisted ultrasound* to improve detection of fetal anomalies (Dunstan et al., 2021).
- *Proteomics* is a promising area that may yield more precise biochemical markers for early pregnancy screening (Norton et al., 2019).

Research gap: Lack of large-scale clinical trials on *AI integration* in prenatal screening.

CONCLUSION

Ultrasound and biochemical screening in pregnancy play complementary roles in prenatal care, helping to detect potential abnormalities early and guide further diagnostic testing. They form a core part of modern obstetric practice, allowing for informed decision-making and better management of pregnancies at risk for complications.

BIBLIOGRAPHY

1. Bianchi DW, Chiu RWK, Lo YMD. Noninvasive prenatal testing: the emergence of a new era in prenatal diagnosis. Prenatal Diagnosis. 2019;39(6):567-75.
2. Gil MM, Quezada MS, Borrell A. Implementation of NIPT in prenatal screening: Evaluation of the detection rate of aneuploidy in high-risk pregnancies. Ultrasound in Obstet Gynecol. 2020;56(2):228-34.
3. Moore JD, Savitz DA, Terry PD. Maternal serum AFP and its role in neural tube defect detection. J Maternal-Fetal and Neonatal Medicine. 2021;34(1):55-62.
4. Nicolaides KH. Screening for fetal anomalies by ultrasound in pregnancy. Am J Obstet Gynecol. 2020;223(5):619-28.
5. Norton ME, Wapner RJ, Kuppermann M. Cell-free DNA analysis for noninvasive examination of trisomy. New Engl J Med. 2019;379(7):715-23.
6. Palomaki GE, Kloza EM, Lambert-Messerlian GM. NIPT versus traditional down syndrome screening in a clinical setting. Genetics in Medicine. 2019;21(1):118-25.
7. Smith GCS, Crossley JA, Aitken DA. Prenatal screening in the first and second trimesters: An integrated approach. J Med Screening. 2022;29(1):25-30.
8. Spencer K, Heath V, Elsheikh A. The quadruple test in down syndrome screening: assessing efficacy. British J Obstet Gynaecol. 2021;128(3):342-9.
9. Tabor A, Madsen M, Obel EB. Invasive testing in pregnancy: balancing risks and benefits. Acta Obstetricia et Gynecologica Scandinavica. 2018;97(6):654-63.
10. Wald NJ, Kennard A, Hackshaw AK. First and second trimester integrated screening for down syndrome. Lancet. 2018;398(5):1379-86.

12

CHAPTER

Rh-negative Pregnancy

Mandakini Pradhan

Q1. When to perform indirect Coombs test?

Draft recommendation:

- RhD-negative woman presenting at first antenatal visit.
- Repeat indirect Coombs test should be done at 28 weeks of gestation before administration of anti-D immune globulin.
- Women presenting with history of HDFN in previous pregnancy irrespective of the RhD status.
- Women with features of hydrops on ultrasonography in present pregnancy irrespective of the RhD status.

Once the indirect Coombs test becomes positive, antibody titers need to be carried out.

Summary of evidence: BCSH Guidelines for Blood Grouping and Red Cell Antibody Testing during pregnancy *(BCSH 2013, NICE 2008)* and *ACOG practice bulletin 2017* both recommend a repeat antibody screen to be performed at 28 weeks of gestation after an initial work-up before first prophylactic anti-D injection is given.

Evidence gap: Larger trials are required determine the need and efficacy of performing indirect Coombs after suspicion of every potential sensitizing event.

Q2. What are the indications of giving injection anti-D?

Draft recommendation:

- Routine anti-Rh(D) prophylaxis during pregnancy is recommended: 1,500 IU (300 µg) at 28–34 weeks.
- For Rh(D)-negative women without prior antibody, i.e., ICT negative delivering a Rh positive newborn is required to be given injection anti-Rh(D) immunoglobulin. Administration of anti-Rh(D) immunoglobulin should be carried out within 72 hours of delivery to women with a Rh(D)-positive newborn, unless already sensitized.
- A dose of 1,500 IU (300 µg) is most recommended. The intramuscular route (in deltoid muscle) is the preferred route. Intravenous route is equally effective if required. The product has to be checked for it.
- Anti-Rh(D) immunoglobulin prophylaxis (100 µg if available, otherwise 300 µg) after a surgical abortion or ectopic pregnancy (all gestational

ages), or after spontaneous or medical abortion/miscarriage after 10 weeks is also recommended.

- Anti-Rh(D) prophylaxis after bleeding, abdominal trauma in pregnancy, and/or fetal death (300 μg) during the second or third trimester must be given. Kleihauer–Betke test can be used to estimate the optimal dose.
- Anti-Rh(D) prophylaxis after amniocentesis, chorionic villus sampling, or external cephalic version must be given.

Summary of evidence: *FIGO 2021* recommends the aforementioned protocol.

ACOG practice bulletin 2017 lists the following as potential sensitizing events in Rh D-negative women in pregnancy:

- Chorionic villus sampling, amniocentesis, cordocentesis
- Threatened miscarriage or miscarriage
- Ectopic pregnancy
- Evacuation of molar pregnancy
- Therapeutic termination of pregnancy
- Antepartum hemorrhage
- Abdominal trauma
- Intrauterine fetal death
- External cephalic version
- Delivery

BCSH 2013 recommends a dose of 250 IU for a sensitizing event prior to 20 weeks, and a dose of 500 IU after 20 weeks for prevention of alloimmunization. Fetomaternal hemorrhage quantification should be done whenever feasible.

Evidence gap: Cost-effectiveness of routine prophylaxis versus calculation of exact dose by FMH quantification using flow cytometry or Kleihauer–Betke test needs to be carried out to prevent inadvertent exposure of RhD negative to plasma regents.

Q3. What are the indications of doing baby blood group using cf DNA test?

Draft recommendation: Noninvasive determination of fetal Rh status is now possible through the analysis of cell-free DNA in maternal plasma. Up to 40% of Rh D negative pregnant women will carry an RhD-negative fetus. In this clinical situation, antenatal anti-D immune globulin administration is unnecessary. Despite the improved accuracy of noninvasive fetal RHD genotyping, cost comparisons with current routine prophylaxis of anti-D immunoglobulin at 28 weeks of gestation have not shown a consistent benefit and are, hence, not recommended at present.

Summary of evidence: Fetal RhD status determination in the first trimester has a sensitivity greater than 99% and a specificity of greater than 95%. *ACOG practice bulletin 2017,* however, raises concerns because of the rate of inconclusive results (range 2–6%), which are influenced by race.

Four cost analyses from North America and Europe have shown no economic benefit at current test-cost levels, whereas a single report from *Canada* suggested it would be cost-effective, although the estimated cost of performing the cell-free DNA was based on a low cost, high-throughput method.

As the cost of this technology diminishes, this may become an attractive and cost-effective strategy. However, at current costs, noninvasive assessment of fetal RhD status is not recommended for routine use at present.

RCOG 2014 recommends to perform fetal genotyping when the antibody reaches a level that would warrant fetal middle cerebral artery (MCA) Doppler monitoring (Level 2 evidence).

Evidence gap: Cost-benefit analysis in Indian settings needs to be carried out to determine the efficacy of using cfDNA for fetal blood group estimation in order to support its implementation.

Q4. What is the indication of doing paternal zygosity testing and what is its relevance in India?

Draft recommendation: In cases of a heterozygous paternal genotype, 50% of the fetuses do not express the involved red cell antigen and, therefore, escape the hemolytic effects of the maternal anti-red cell antibody. In these cases, further maternal and fetal testing can be eliminated. However, cost comparisons with current routine prophylaxis of anti-D immunoglobulin at 28 weeks of gestation have not shown a consistent benefit and, thus, this test is not routinely recommended.

Summary of evidence: Most red cell antigens are inherited through codominant alleles. As an example, for the E/e antigen, an individual can be homozygous E/E, homozygous e/e, or heterozygous E/e. This is not the case, however, for RhD, as there is no "d" antigen because it represents a gene deletion and a lack of translation to a protein. In the case of RhD, quantitative polymerase chain reaction can be used to test for the number of copies of the D gene by comparing the DNA peak to that of the RHCE gene, which is always present as two copies in all individuals. However, *RCOG green top guideline 2014* deems it reasonable to omit paternal testing and proceed directly to fetal genotyping, when feasible, to avoid issues of nonpaternity.

Evidence gap: Cost-benefit analysis in Indian settings needs to be carried out to determine the efficacy of doing paternal zygosity testing in order to support its implementation.

Q5. How do we monitor Rh isoimmunized pregnancy?

Draft recommendation:

- Low antibody titers of 1:2–1:4 may indicate the antibody response from previous anti-D injection. Antibody titers less than critical titers need to be repeated at 2–3 weekly till 28 weeks of gestation and then 2 weekly until delivery.
- Antibody titers greater than critical titers (>1:8 or 1:16, depending upon the laboratory cut-offs) need to be followed up with serial middle cerebral artery Doppler monitoring every 1–2 weeks. Titers need not be repeated after crossing of critical tires.
- Once middle cerebral artery Doppler shows a peak systolic velocity (PSV) of >1.5 MoM, it is strongly indicative of fetal anemia and referral to fetal medicine specialist for determining the need for intrauterine transfusion needs to be carried out.

Summary of evidence: *RCOG green top guideline, 2014* strongly recommends (Level 2 evidence) to ascertain the cause of the alloimmunization: for example, inadequate or omitted anti-D prophylaxis or a previous blood transfusion. Details of previously affected pregnancies, particularly IUTs and the gestation at which they were commenced, neonatal anemia, gestation at delivery, and the need for exchange transfusions or phototherapy, should also be obtained. This information enables a risk assessment of the pregnancy to be made. Ultrasound monitoring should commence once there is a moderate or severe risk of fetal anemia.

ACOG practice bulletin, 2018 says (level 2 evidence) that MCA PSV monitoring is predictive of moderate or severe fetal anemia with 100% sensitivity and a false positive rate of 12%.

Evidence gap: Use of middle cerebral artery Doppler for monitoring of fetal anemia after 34–35 weeks of gestation is controversial due to its decreasing sensitivity and increase in false positive rates. Monitoring strategy in such cases needs to be implored upon.

Q6. What are the conditions in which multiple anti-D injections may be required?

Draft recommendation:

- Suspected large fetomaternal hemorrhage as in cases of abruptio placentae/ongoing antenatal hemorrhage
- Intrauterine fetal death with abruptio placentae
- RhD-negative women of childbearing potential receiving D positive blood/blood products

After the calculation of the amount of fetomaternal hemorrhage using Kleihauer–Betke test or flow cytometry, 1,500 IU of injection anti-D is given for every 30 mL of FMH. Intramuscular injections every 12 hours until the desired dose or intravascular administration of 3,000 IU every 8 hourly until the total desired dose can be given.

Summary of evidence:

Ongoing antenatal hemorrhage: ACOG practice bulletin 2017 recommends anti-D immune globulin for Rh D-negative women who experience antenatal hemorrhage after 20 weeks of gestation. The volume of fetal-maternal hemorrhage needs to be assessed with a quantitative test (such as the Kleihauer-Betke test). The appropriate amount of RhD immune globulin should then be administered to cover the estimated volume of fetal-maternal hemorrhage. In cases of chronic or episodic bleeding, this approach may need to be repeated. Another strategy is to monitor the RhD-negative patient with continuing antenatal hemorrhage with serial indirect Coombs testing for anti-D approximately every 3 weeks. If the result is positive, indicating the persistence of anti-D immune globulin, then theoretically no additional treatment with anti-D immune globulin is necessary.

If the Coombs test result is negative, excessive fetal-maternal hemorrhage may have occurred, and a Kleihauer-Betke test should be performed in order to determine the amount of additional anti-D immune globulin necessary.

BCSH 2013 recommends a dose of 500 IU every 6 weeks for continuing uterine bleeding. In the event of intermittent uterine bleeding, they recommend estimation of fetal-maternal hemorrhage be carried out at 2-weekly intervals.

Intrauterine fetal death: *BCSH 2013* recommends if there is an intrauterine death (IUD) and no sample can be obtained from the baby, prophylactic anti-D Ig should be administered to D-negative, previously nonsensitized women. A minimum of 500 IU of anti-D Ig should be administered within 72 h following the diagnosis of IUD. Maternal samples should be tested for FMH and additional dose(s) given as guided by FMH tests. It should be noted that the diagnosis of IUD is the sensitizing event rather than delivery and hence anti-D Ig should be administered within 72 h of diagnosis.

D-positive platelet transfusions: A dose of 250 IU anti-D immunoglobulin is recommended by *BCSH 2013* to cover up to five adult therapeutic doses of D-positive platelets given within a 6-week period.

Inadvertent transfusion of D-positive blood to D-negative women: Injection anti-D 1,500 or 2,500 IU IV or IM is recommended by *BSCH 2013;* however, IV anti-D immunoglobulin is the preparation of choice, achieving adequate plasma levels immediately. The quantitation of D positive red cells should be performed by flow cytometry after 48 h if an IV dose of anti-D has been given or 72 h if an IM dose has been given, and further anti-D Ig given until there are no detectable D positive red cells in circulation. When more than one unit of D positive blood has been transfused, a red cell exchange transfusion should be considered to reduce the load of D positive red cells in the circulation and the dose of anti-D Ig required to prevent immunization.

A single blood-volume red cell exchange transfusion will achieve a 65–70% reduction in D-positive red cells; a double volume exchange will achieve an 85–90% reduction. Shortly after the exchange transfusion, the residual volume of D positive red cells should be estimated using flow cytometry.

Evidence gap: Anti-D appears to persist in most patients for 12 weeks. More research is needed to determine the frequency of repeating injection anti-D in cases where there is continual uterine bleeding keeping in mind the cost of treatment in resource-limited settings.

Q7. What is the timing of delivery in RhD-negative pregnancies?

Draft recommendation:

- *RhD-negative nonisoimmunized pregnancy:* Induction of labor at 40 weeks.
- *Mild fetal hemolysis (red cell antibodies present which can cause fetal anemia but have remained stable throughout pregnancy):* Induction of labor at 37–38 weeks of gestation.
- *Severely sensitized pregnancies requiring intrauterine transfusions:* Fetal medicine team in collaboration with neonatal intensive care unit makes decisions about the adequate timing of delivery of these pregnancies. The aim is to time the delivery such as to ensure that the fetus is not significantly anemic at birth.

Summary of evidence: In severely anemic fetuses, *ACOG practice bulletin 2018* suggests—last transfusion be performed at 30–32 weeks of gestation, with delivery at 32–34 weeks of gestation after maternal steroid administration to enhance fetal pulmonary maturity. In a review of 281 pregnancies by *Boggs* et al., it is recommended that intrauterine transfusions be performed up to 36 weeks of gestation when feasible in order to limit neonatal morbidity. In such cases, delivery can then be accomplished between 37 and 38 weeks of gestation.

Evidence gap: There is wide variation in recommendation for optimal timing of delivery in patients receiving intrauterine transfusions. More research in needed in this area.

BIBLIOGRAPHY

1. American College of Obstetricians and Gynecologists. ACOG practice bulletin No. 181: Prevention of Rh D Alloimmunization. Obstet Gynecol. 2017;130(2):e57-e70.

2. American College of Obstetricians and Gynecologists. ACOG practice bulletin No. 192: Management of alloimmunization during pregnancy. Obstet Gynecol. 2018;131(3):e82-e90.
3. Qureshi H, Massey E, Kirwan D, et al. British Committee for standards in haematology guideline for the use of anti-D immunoglobulin for the prevention of haemolytic disease of the fetus and newborn. Transfus Med. 2014;24(1):8-20.
4. RCOG. RCOG green top guideline no. 65: The Management of Women with Red Cell Antibodies during Pregnancy. [online] Available from https://www.rcog.org.uk/guidance/browse-all-guidance/green-top-guidelines/the-management-of-women-with-red-cell-antibodies-during-pregnancy-green-top-guideline-no-65/. [Last accessed November, 2024].
5. Visser GHA, Thommesen T, Di Renzo GC, et al. FIGO/ICM guidelines for preventing Rhesus disease: a call to action. Int J Gynaecol Obstet. 2021;152(2):144-7.

13

CHAPTER

Draft Guideline for Electronic Fetal Monitoring

Vandana Bansal, Meera Agalawe

INTRODUCTION

Continuous electronic fetal heart monitoring (EFM) in labor was introduced in 1970s to identify events that might result in hypoxic ischemic encephalopathy, cerebral palsy, or fetal death, and was quickly adopted by most obstetricians and obstetric societies as a significant improvement in intrapartum fetal care. The purpose of fetal monitoring in labor was to recognize these fetuses which might be at risk of hypoxic injury so that delivery can be expedited and perinatal outcomes improved. On the other hand, accurate identification of appropriately oxygenated fetuses would prevent unnecessary interventions.

The use of EFM has grown dramatically in laboring pregnant women making it the most common obstetric procedure. Electronic fetal monitoring (EFM) or cardiotocography (CTG) is the current mainstay of intrapartum fetal monitoring worldwide. However, the benefits of this intervention have not been conclusively demonstrated.

Q1. Intermittent auscultation versus electronic fetal monitoring in labor?

Draft recommendations:

- Intermittent auscultation is equivalent to continuous EFM in screening for fetal compromise in low-risk patients. Cardiotocography may be performed continuously or in an intermittent manner.
- Structured intermittent auscultation may be carried out using a Pinard stethoscope or a handheld Doppler machine. Intermittent auscultation is performed every 15 minutes in the first stage of labor and with every contraction or every 5 minutes in the second stage of labor for a duration of 60 seconds. Auscultation should be commenced immediately after a palpable uterine contraction and continued for 1 minute after the contraction has ended.
- Continuous EFM should be used when there are abnormalities in structured intermittent auscultation or for high-risk patients
- Antenatal initial risk assessment should be done at onset of labor to decide need for structured intermittent auscultation or continuous electronic fetal monitoring.
- The potential benefits and risks of continuous EFM and structured intermittent auscultation should be discussed during prenatal care and

labor, and a decision reached by the pregnant woman and her physician, with the understanding that if intrapartum clinical situations warrant, continuous EFM may be recommended.

Evidence: As per the American College of Obstetrics and Gynecology (ACOG 2009), Intermittent auscultation or continuous electronic monitoring is considered acceptable method of intrapartum surveillance in low-risk pregnancies.

The National Institute for Health and Care Excellence (NICE 2022) gives strict criteria for Structured Intermittent auscultation which is defined as measurement of the fetal heart rate at regular intervals from the time of admission of the patient till delivery. However, the safety in using structured intermittent auscultation is based on a nurse-to-patient ratio of 1:1.

Gaps in literature: Despite the widespread use, the limitations of EFM include poor interobserver and intraobserver reliability, uncertain efficacy, and a high false-positive rate. There is a risk of increased intervention with continuous CTG monitoring compared to intermittent auscultation which may outweigh the benefits. It may also restrict her mobility and the option of labor under water (NICE guideline).

Q2. Does intrapartum electronic fetal monitoring reduce perinatal morbidity and mortality?

Draft recommendations:

- For both low- and high-risk pregnancies, continuous electronic FHR monitoring is not clearly superior to intermittent auscultation with respect to preventing fetal death or poor long-term neurologic outcome in the newborn and has a high false-positive rate.
- There has been no demonstrable reduction in the overall perinatal mortality rate, incidence of cerebral palsy or cord blood acidosis with continuous cardiotocography as compared to intermittent auscultation. Continuous cardiotocography, however, has been associated with halving of neonatal seizures rate.
- There is evidence that the use of EFM increases the rate of cesarean deliveries and operative vaginal deliveries secondary to erroneous diagnosis of fetal distress in electronically monitored patients (high false positive rate). These limitations are due to high inter-observer and intraobserver variability which may play a major role in interpretation.
- In spite of all these shortcomings, electronic fetal monitoring provides the obstetricians information with high degree of reliability about both extremes, i.e., presence of fetal wellbeing (normal FHR pattern), as well as presence of severe fetal problems (pathological FHR).

Evidence: The rate of cerebral palsy has essentially remained the same since World War II despite fetal monitoring, advancements in treatments and interventions.

A 2017 meta-analysis of 13 randomized trials in >37,000 low- and high-risk pregnancies that compared continuous electronic FHR monitoring with intermittent auscultation reported the following major findings:

No statistically significant differences between techniques were noted for the following newborn/childhood outcomes:

- Acidemia (measured in cord blood)
- Apgar score <4 at five minutes
- Neonatal intensive care unit admission
- Hypoxic-ischemic encephalopathy
- Perinatal mortality
- Neurodevelopmental impairment at ≥12 months of age
- Cerebral palsy

Although use of continuous electronic FHR monitoring resulted in fewer neonatal seizures, there were no differences in long-term neurologic outcomes.

Continuous electronic FHR monitoring resulted in:

- More operative vaginal births for abnormal FHR patterns or acidosis
- Fewer spontaneous vaginal births
- More cesarean births for abnormal FHR patterns or acidosis
- More operative vaginal and cesarean births overall

However, these studies were carried out in the 1970s, 1980s, and early 1990s where equipment, clinical experience, and interpretation criteria were very different from current practice, and they were clearly underpowered to evaluate differences in major outcomes.

It is important to note that all seven trials published after 1980 found no significant increase in the rate of cesarean birth for patients monitored continuously compared with those monitored by intermittent auscultation, in contrast to the four small trials published before 1980, which found significantly higher rates of cesarean birth with continuous monitoring.

It is also important to note that a statistical reduction in the perinatal death rate with continuous intrapartum FHR monitoring is difficult to demonstrate because death is a rare outcome. Even the pooled results from multiple randomized trials lacked sufficient power to permit a definitive conclusion in the 2017 meta-analysis.

However, a previous meta-analysis that specifically evaluated perinatal deaths attributed to fetal hypoxia in low- and high-risk pregnancies concluded that this outcome was significantly less common in continuously monitored patients than those monitored with intermittent auscultation (7/9398 versus 17/9163; 0.7 versus 1.8 per 1000; odds ratio 0.41, 95% CI 0.17-0.98; nine trials).

A statistical reduction in the incidence of cerebral palsy with continuous intrapartum FHR monitoring is also difficult to prove for several reasons. Many cases of cerebral palsy are due to antepartum, rather than intrapartum, events. In such cases, intrapartum interventions are unlikely to change the course of the disease. In addition, most FHR abnormalities are not associated with fetal acidemia or hypoxemia, and most fetal acidemia and hypoxemia do not result in neurologic disability. Another potentially confounding factor is that a pre-existing fetal neurologic disorder may be the cause, rather than the result, of an intrapartum FHR abnormality.

A more recent 2021 network meta-analysis (33 trials, >118,000 participants) evaluated multiple forms of intrapartum fetal monitoring, including intermittent auscultation and cardiotocography with and without computer-aided decision support, fetal scalp lactate assessment, fetal scalp pH analysis, fetal pulse oximetry, and fetal ST segment analysis (STAN). No method of intrapartum fetal monitoring increased or decreased the overall cesarean birth rate or clinical outcomes. Compared with other forms of intrapartum fetal monitoring, intermittent auscultation neither reduced nor increased adverse neonatal outcomes, including low Apgar scores, neonatal acidemia, neonatal intensive care unit admissions, or perinatal deaths. Intermittent auscultation was associated with fewer emergency cesarean births overall and fewer emergency cesarean births for fetal distress.

The risk-benefit debate will continue to focus on cesarean section and neonatal seizures. Given the perceived conflict between the risk for the mother (increased cesarean section and instrumental vaginal delivery rate) and benefit for the baby (decreased incidence of neonatal seizures), it is difficult to make quality judgments about which effect is more important.

Q3. Which are the high-risk pregnancies which require continuous monitoring in labor?

Draft recommendations: Antenatal high-risk factors for fetal compromise identified before the onset of labor requiring continuous EFM may be maternal or fetal factors and include:

- *Maternal risk factors:*
    - Medical disorders like hypertensive disorder, preexisting diabetes (type 1 or 2) and gestational diabetes requiring medications, chronic renal disease, cyanotic heart disease, autoimmune disorders, and thrombophilia
    - Antepartum hemorrhage
    - Previous LSCS or other full thickness uterine scar
    - Prolonged pregnancy >42 weeks
- *Fetal risk factors:*
    - Oligohydramnios or polyhydramnios

- Abnormal umbilical artery Doppler
- Multiple pregnancy
- Prematurity
- Fetal growth restriction (estimated fetal weight <3rd centile)
- Small for gestational age (EFW/AC 3rd to 10th centile) with abnormal Doppler ultrasound, oligohydramnios and falling centiles on growth graphs

▪ A low-risk pregnancy may be reclassified as a high-risk pregnancy at any time before or during the process of labor. Intrapartum factors necessitating continuous EFM include:
  - Abnormal admission test
  - Meconium stained liquor
  - Abnormal fetal heart on auscultation
  - Maternal pyrexia (a temperature of 38°C or above on a single reading or 37.5°C or above on 2 consecutive occasions 1 hour apart)
  - Suspected chorioamnionitis
  - Fresh vaginal bleeding more than show that develops in labor
  - Blood stained liquor that may indicate suspected antepartum hemorrhage
  - Prolonged rupture of membranes
  - Induced or augmented labor with the probability of excessive uterine activity
  - Epidural/regional analgesia
  - Reduced fetal movements in the previous 24 hours of onset of labor
  - Delay in the first or second stage of labor
  - Contractions that last longer than 2 minutes, or 5 or more contractions in 10 minutes
  - Hypertension that developed in labor

If continuous cardiotocography was used because of concerns arising from intermittent auscultation but the tracing is normal after 20 minutes of observation, the cardiotocograph can be removed and return to intermittent auscultation can be offered.

Evidence: FIGO consensus guidelines on intrapartum fetal monitoring suggests that although the studies are controversial for its use in low risk pregnancies, continuous CTG monitoring should be considered in all situations where there is a high risk of fetal hypoxia/acidosis, whether due to maternal health conditions (such as vaginal hemorrhage and maternal pyrexia), abnormal fetal growth during pregnancy, epidural analgesia, meconium stained liquor, or the possibility of excessive uterine activity, as occurs with induced or augmented labor. Continuous CTG is also recommended when abnormalities are detected during intermittent fetal auscultation. NICE in its 2022 amendment also suggests offering continuous

CTG monitoring as part of fetal assessment if any antenatal or intrapartum risk factors for fetal compromise are present.

Q4. Which classification scheme/categorization should be used for interpreting and decision making with regards to electronic fetal monitor tracings in labor?

Draft recommendations:

- Any of the method of classifying CTG whether it is the Three-Tiered Fetal Heart Rate Interpretation System by ACOG which is similar to FIGO consensus guidelines or the new updated guidelines by the NICE can be used for clinical practice.
- To provide a systematic approach to interpreting the electronic fetal monitor tracing, the National Institute of Child Health and Human Development convened a workshop in 2008 to revise the accepted definitions for electronic fetal monitor tracing. The key elements include assessment of baseline heart rate, presence or absence of variability, and interpretation of periodic changes. The workshop introduced a new classification scheme for decision making with regard to tracings. The objective of the guidelines was to reduce the inconsistent use of common terminology and the wide variability that sometimes occurs in FHR interpretations. ACOG guidelines issued in 2009 supported the recommendations of the Eunice Kennedy Shriver National Institute of Child and Health Development workshop on electronic fetal monitoring. This was followed by more international guidelines including the FIGO consensus guidelines on Intrapartum fetal monitoring in 2015 and the NICE guideline of fetal monitoring in labor recently updated in 2022. All the International practice guidelines on electronic intrapartum fetal monitoring are essentially trying to describe the characteristics similarly with some essential variations.

Evidence:

Electronic fetal monitoring: Characteristics of the parameter assessed.

Pattern	*Definition*
Baseline heart rate	• The mean FHR rounded to increments of 5 beats per minute during a 10-minute segment, excluding accelerations and decelerations or periods of marked FHR variability • The baseline must be stable for a minimum of 2 minutes in any 10-minute segment, or the baseline for that time period is indeterminate. In that case, one may refer to the prior 10-minute window for determination of baseline. When deciding if there is any change in baseline fetal heart rate, compare it with earlier CTG traces • *Normal FHR baseline:* 110–160 beats per minute

Contd...

Contd...

Pattern	***Definition***
	• *Tachycardia:* FHR baseline is greater than 160 beats per minute • *Bradycardia:* FHR baseline is less than 110 beats per minute Preterm fetuses tend to have values toward the upper end of this range and post-term fetuses towards the lower end
Baseline variability	• Fluctuations in the baseline FHR that are irregular in amplitude and frequency in a one minute segment of the trace between contractions excluding decelerations and accelerations • Variability is visually quantitated as the amplitude of peak-to-trough in beats per minute and normal variability is 5–25 bpm – Absent—amplitude range undetectable – Minimal/reduced—amplitude range detectable but less than 5 beats per minute – Moderate (normal)—amplitude range 5–25 beats per minute – —Marked/saltatory/increased—amplitude range greater than 25 beats per minute
Acceleration	• A visually apparent abrupt increase (onset to peak in less than 30 seconds) in the FHR • At 32 weeks of gestation and beyond, an acceleration has a peak of 15 beats per minute or more above baseline, with a duration of 15 seconds or more but less than 2 minutes from onset to return • Before 32 weeks of gestation, an acceleration has a peak of 10 beats per minute or more above baseline, with a duration of 10 seconds or more but less than 2 minutes from onset to return • Prolonged acceleration lasts 2 minutes or more but less than 10 minutes in duration • If an acceleration lasts 10 minutes or longer, it is a baseline change
Early deceleration	• Visually apparent usually symmetrical gradual decrease and return of the FHR associated with a uterine contraction of more than 15 bpm in amplitude, and lasting more than 15 seconds • A gradual FHR decrease is defined as from the onset to the FHR nadir of 30 seconds or more • The nadir of the deceleration occurs at the same time as the peak of the contraction • In most cases, the onset, nadir, and recovery of the deceleration are coincident with the beginning, peak, and ending of the contraction, respectively
Late deceleration	• Visually apparent usually symmetrical gradual decrease and return of the FHR associated with a uterine contraction • The deceleration is delayed in timing, with the nadir of the deceleration occurring after the peak of the contraction • In most cases, the onset, nadir, and recovery of the deceleration occur after the beginning, peak, and ending of the contraction, respectively

Contd...

Contd...

Pattern	Definition
	Described by FIGO as U-shaped and/or with reduced variability with decelerations with a gradual onset and/or a gradual return to the baseline and/or reduced variability within the deceleration
Variable deceleration	• Visually apparent abrupt decrease in FHR • An abrupt FHR decrease is defined as from the onset of the deceleration to the beginning of the FHR nadir of less than 30 seconds • The decrease in FHR is 15 beats per minute or greater, lasting 15 seconds or greater, and less than 2 minutes in duration • When variable decelerations are associated with uterine contractions, their onset, depth, and duration commonly vary with successive uterine contractions *FIGO describes it as (V-shaped):* Decelerations that exhibit a rapid drop (onset to nadir in less than 30 seconds), good variability within the deceleration, rapid recovery to the baseline, varying size, shape, and relationship to uterine contractions
Prolonged deceleration	• Visually apparent decrease in the FHR below the baseline • Decrease in FHR from the baseline that is 15 beats per minute or more, lasting 2 minutes or more but less than 10 minutes in duration (FIGO suggests a duration of 3 minutes) • If a deceleration lasts 10 minutes or longer, it is a baseline change
Sinusoidal pattern	Visually apparent, smooth, sine wave-like undulating pattern in FHR baseline with a cycle frequency of 3–5 per minute which persists for 20 minutes or more

Guidelines for nomenclature and interpretation of electronic fetal heart rate monitoring: As per the updated NICE guidelines, all 4 features of the cardiotocography trace (contractions, baseline fetal heart rate, variability, decelerations) should then be categorize as white, amber or red (indicating increasing levels of concern) and use alongside consideration of the presence of accelerations to classify the overall CTG trace.

Contractions: It is important to assess the pressure tracing before assessing the fetal tracing to accurately interpret decelerations. The electronic fetal monitor uses an external pressure transducer to measure frequency, basal tone, and duration of contractions. However, the strength of contractions cannot always be accurately assessed from an external transducer. Uterine contractions are quantified as the number of contractions present in a 10-minute window, averaged over a 30-minute period.

Normal or white: Five contractions or less in 10 minutes, averaged over a 30-minute window.

Tachysystole or amber: More than five contractions in 10 minutes, averaged over a 30-minute window. Tachysystole should always be qualified as to the presence or absence of associated FHR decelerations.

The term tachysystole applies to both spontaneous and stimulated labor. The clinical response to tachysystole may differ depending on whether contractions are spontaneous or stimulated. The terms hyperstimulation and hypercontractility have been abandoned.

Baseline heart rate: Stable baseline of 110 to 160 beats a minute is considered normal or white.

Mild bradycardia (100 to 110 bpm) is associated with post-term infants and occipitoposterior position. Although a baseline fetal heart rate between 100 and 109 beats a minute is an amber feature, continue usual care if this has been stable throughout labor and there is normal variability and no variable or late decelerations.

Rates of less than 100 bpm are considered as red feature and may be seen in fetuses with congenital heart disease, myocardial conduction defects, drugs like beta-blockers and narcotics or maternal hypotension.

A baseline greater than 160 bpm is defined as tachycardia and is a red feature. This is associated with certain maternal and fetal conditions, such as chorioamnionitis, hypoxia, fever, dehydration, drugs like beta-mimetics and tachyarrhythmias.

Variability: The FHR normally exhibits variability, with an average change of 5 to 25 bpm of the baseline rate and is characterized as white, and is linked to the fetal central nervous system. Therefore, it is a vital clue in determining the overall fetal condition. The NICHD has stated that it is no longer useful to distinguish between short-term and long-term variability and has categorized variability into absent, minimal, moderate and marked. Sleep cycles of 20 to 40 minutes or longer may cause a normal decrease in FHR variability, as can certain medications, including analgesics, anesthetics, barbiturates, and magnesium sulfate. Loss or reduction of variability, accompanied by other CTG changes particularly rise in baseline heart rate or late or variable decelerations, increases the possibility of fetal compromise if uncorrected.

Fewer than 5 beats a minute for between 30 and 50 minutes, or more than 25 beats a minute for up to 10 minutes is categorized as amber.

Isolated reduction in variability to fewer than 5 beats per minute for more than 30 minutes when combined with antenatal or intrapartum risk factors should be reviewed and considered for expediting delivery as this is associated with an increased risk of adverse neonatal outcomes.

If there is a reduction in variability to fewer than 5 beats per minute combined with other CTG changes, particularly a rise in the baseline fetal heart rate, as this is a strong indicator for fetal compromise.

If the duration of decreased variability extends to more than 50 minutes or increased variability of more than 25 bpm for more than 10 minutes or sinusoidal pattern, it is designated as red.

Absence of variability is a very concerning feature and is designated as red and it must be reviewed in context of the whole clinical picture with a low threshold for expedited birth.

Sinusoidal pattern is a smooth, undulating sine wave pattern defined by an amplitude of 10 bpm with three to five cycles per minute, lasting at least 20 minutes. This uncommon pattern is associated with severe fetal anemia and hydrops, and it usually requires rapid intervention in these settings. Similar appearing benign tracings occasionally occur because of "fetal thumb sucking" or maternal narcotic administration, and generally these will persist for less than 10 minutes.

Accelerations: Abrupt increases in the FHR are associated with fetal movement or stimulation and are indicative of fetal wellbeing. The presence of fetal heart rate accelerations, even with reduced variability, is generally a sign that the baby is healthy. On the other hand, absence of accelerations on an otherwise normal CTG trace does not indicate fetal acidosis.

Decelerations: Decelerations are transient episodes when the fetal heart rate slows to below the baseline level by more than 15 beats a minute, with each episode lasting 15 seconds or more. The decrease in FHR is calculated from the onset to the nadir of the deceleration. They are described as early, variable, and late in relation to uterine contractions. Decelerations are classified as recurrent if they occur with 50 percent or more of contractions in a 20-minute period, and intermittent if they occur with less than 50 percent of contractions.

The significance of decelerations in fetal heart rate must be assessed in relation to:

- Their timing (early, variable or late) in relation to the peaks and duration of the contractions
- The duration of the individual decelerations
- Whether or not the fetal heart rate returns to the baseline
- How long they have been present for
- Whether they occur with over 50% of contractions (defined as repetitive/ recurrent)
- The presence or absence of shouldering
- The variability within the deceleration

The longer and later the individual decelerations, the higher the risk of fetal compromise (particularly if the decelerations are accompanied by a rise in the baseline, a tachycardia, or reduced or increased variability).

Early decelerations are transient, gradual decreases in FHR that are visually apparent and usually symmetric. They occur with and mirror the uterine contraction and seldom go below 100 bpm.

The nadir of the deceleration occurs at the same time as the peak of the contraction. Early decelerations are nearly always benign and probably indicate head compression, which is a normal part of labor. They are not accompanied by any other CTG changes, such as reduced variability or a rise in the baseline fetal heart rate.

Variable decelerations, as the name implies, vary in terms of shape, depth, and timing in relationship to uterine contractions, but they are visually apparent, abrupt decreases in FHR. Characteristics of variable decelerations include rapid descent and recovery, good baseline variability, and accelerations at the onset and at the end of the contraction (i.e., "shoulders"). When they are associated with uterine contractions, their onset, depth, and duration commonly vary with successive uterine contractions. Overall, variable decelerations are usually benign, and their physiologic basis is usually related to cord compression, with subsequent changes in peripheral vascular resistance or oxygenation. They occur especially in the second stage of labor, when cord compression is most common. Atypical variable decelerations may indicate fetal hypoxemia, with characteristic features that include late onset (in relation to contractions), loss of shoulders, and slow recovery.

If variable decelerations persist and other CTG changes are present, there is a risk of fetal compromise and acidosis. Start conservative measures and carry out an urgent obstetric review if there are decelerations lasting longer than 30 minutes in the presence of either a rise in the baseline heart rate or reduced variability. Take into account antenatal and intrapartum risk factors, such as suspected sepsis, the presence of meconium, slow progress of labor or the use of oxytocin, to determine whether there is a need for expedited birth.

Characteristics of variable decelerations which are of concern (previously called as atypical variable decelerations):

- Lasting more than 60 seconds
- Reduced variability within the deceleration
- Failure or slow return to baseline fetal heart rate
- Loss of previously present shouldering

Variable decelerations with no concerning characteristics and no other CTG changes (previously called as typical variable decelerations), including no rise in the baseline fetal heart rate can be a normal feature in an otherwise uncomplicated labor and birth, and are usually a result of cord compression. In such situation support the woman to change position or mobilize.

Late decelerations are visually apparent, usually symmetric, and have the characteristic feature of onset of the deceleration after the onset of the uterine contraction. The timing of the deceleration is delayed, with the nadir of the deceleration occurring after the peak of the contraction.

The physiology behind late deceleration is uteroplacental insufficiency. Transient late deceleration patterns may be seen with maternal hypotension or uterine hyperstimulation.

The longer and later the individual decelerations, the higher the risk of fetal compromise (particularly if the decelerations are accompanied by a rise in the baseline, a tachycardia or reduced or increased variability).

Prolonged decelerations last longer than two minutes, but less than 10 minutes. They may be caused by a number of factors, including head compression (rapid fetal descent), cord compression, or uteroplacental insufficiency. Management depends on the clinical picture and presence of other FHR characteristics.

To categorize these decelerations the NICE updated guidelines recommend assigning the color as follows:
White:

- No decelerations, or
- Early decelerations, or
- Variable decelerations that are not evolving to have concerning

Amber:

- Repetitive variable decelerations with any concerning characteristics for less than 30 minutes, or
- Variable decelerations with any concerning characteristics for more than 30 minutes, or
- Repetitive late decelerations for less than 30 minutes

Red:

- Repetitive variable decelerations with any concerning characteristics for more than 30 minutes, or
- Repetitive late decelerations for more than 30 minutes, or
- Acute bradycardia, or a single prolonged deceleration lasting 3 minutes or

Categorization of cardiotocography traces (all stages of labor):
Overall assessment: The recommendations for the overall management of FHR tracings by NICHD, the International Federation of Gynecology and Obstetrics, and ACOG agree that interpretation is reproducible at the extreme ends of the fetal monitor strip spectrum. For example, the presence of a normal baseline rate with FHR accelerations or moderate variability predicts the absence of fetal acidemia. Bradycardia, absence of variability and accelerations, and presence of recurrent late or variable decelerations may predict current or impending fetal asphyxia. However, more than 50 percent of fetal strips fall between these two extremes, in which overall recommendations cannot be made reliably. In the 2008 revision of the NICHD, a three-tiered system for the categorization of FHR patterns was recommended and adopted by

ACOG: normal (category I), indeterminate (category II), and abnormal (category III). Category III tracings need intervention to resolve the abnormal tracing or to move toward expeditious delivery.

Classification of fetal heart rate tracings as per ACOG: It is important to recognize that FHR tracing patterns provide information only on the current acid-base status of the fetus. Categorization of the FHR tracing evaluates the fetus at that point in time. An FHR tracing may move back and forth between the categories depending on the clinical situation and management strategies used.

Category I: FHR tracings are normal. Category I FHR tracings are strongly predictive of normal fetal acid-base status at the time of observation. Category I FHR tracings may be monitored in a routine manner, and no specific action is required.

Category II: FHR tracings are indeterminate. Category II FHR tracings are not predictive of abnormal fetal acid-base status, yet presently there is not adequate evidence to classify these as Category I or Category III. Category II FHR tracings require evaluation and continued surveillance and reevaluation, taking into account the entire associated clinical circumstances. In some circumstances, either ancillary tests to ensure fetal wellbeing or intrauterine resuscitative measures may be used with Category II tracings.

Category III: FHR tracings are abnormal. Category III tracings are associated with abnormal fetal acid-base status at the time of observation. Category III FHR tracings require prompt evaluation. Depending on the clinical situation, efforts to expeditiously resolve the abnormal FHR pattern may include but are not limited to provision of maternal oxygen, change in maternal position, discontinuation of labor stimulation, treatment of maternal hypotension, and treatment of tachysystole with FHR changes. If a Category III tracing does not resolve with these measures, delivery should be undertaken.

Three-tiered fetal heart rate interpretation system:

Category I:

Category I FHR tracings include all of the following:

- *Baseline rate:* 110–160 beats per minute
- *Baseline FHR variability:* Moderate
- *Late or variable decelerations:* Absent
- *Early decelerations:* Present or absent
- *Accelerations:* Present or absent

Category II:

Category II FHR tracings include all FHR tracings not categorized as Category I or Category III. Category II tracings may represent an appreciable fraction of those encountered in clinical care. Examples of Category II FHR tracings include any of the following:

Contd...

Contd...

Baseline rate
- Bradycardia not accompanied by absent baseline variability
- Tachycardia

Baseline FHR variability
- Minimal baseline variability
- Absent baseline variability with no recurrent decelerations
- Marked baseline variability

Accelerations
Absence of induced accelerations after fetal stimulation

Periodic or episodic decelerations
- Recurrent variable decelerations accompanied by minimal or moderate baseline variability
- Prolonged deceleration more than 2 minutes but less than 10 minutes
- Recurrent late decelerations with moderate baseline variability
- Variable decelerations with other characteristics such as slow return to baseline, overshoots, or "shoulders"

Category III:
Category III FHR tracings include either:
- Absent baseline FHR variability and any of the following:
  - Recurrent late decelerations
  - Recurrent variable decelerations
  - Bradycardia
- Sinusoidal pattern

Categorization of cardiotocography traces as per NICE guidelines: CTG traces are categorized based on whether each of the 4 features (contractions, baseline, variability, decelerations) have been scored as white, amber, or red:

Definition of normal, suspicious, and pathological FHR traces:

Normal: A FHR trace in which all four features are classified as reassuring (all four features white)
Suspicious: An FHR trace with one feature classified as non-reassuring/amber and the remaining features classified as reassuring
Pathological: An FHR trace with two or more features classified as non-reassuring/amber or one or more classified as abnormal/red

Category definition:

Features	***Baseline (bpm)***	***Variability (bpm)***	***Deceleration***	***Acceleration***
Reassuring (white)	110–160	5–25 bpm	• None • Early decelerations • Variable deceleration with no concerning characteristics (typical variable)	Present
Nonreassuring (Amber)	• 100–109 or • Increase in baseline fetal heart rate of 20 beats a minute or more from the start of labor or since the last review an hour ago • Unable to determine baseline	• <5 for • 30–50 minutes • More than 25 beats a minute for up to 10 minutes	• Repetitive variable decelerations with concerning characteristics (in over 50% of contractions), occurring for less than 30 minutes • Variable decelerations with concerning characteristics for more than 30 minutes • Repetitive late decelerations for less than 30 minutes	The absence of accelerations with otherwise normal trace does not indicate fetal acidosis
Abnormal (Red)	<100 >160	• <5 for more than 50 minutes • More than 25 beats a minute for more than 10 minutes • Sinusoidal • pattern ≥10 minutes	• Repetitive variable • Decelerations with concerning characteristics for more than 30 minutes • Repetitive late decelerations for more than 30 minutes • Single prolonged • deceleration for more than 3 minutes • Acute bradycardia	

Management as per CTG category: If CTG trace categorized as suspicious and there are no other concerning risk factors, do a full clinical assessment and manage conservatively. However, if the CTG is suspicious and there are additional intrapartum risk factors such as slow progress, sepsis, or meconium, do a full clinical assessment and undertake conservative measures and consider fetal scalp stimulation or expedite delivery.

If CTG trace categorized as pathological exclude acute events (cord prolapse, suspected placental abruption or suspected uterine rupture) that need immediate intervention. Do a full clinical assessment, undertake conservative measures and if the CTG is still pathological, consider expediting birth.

- If repeated accelerations are present with reduced variability, the FHR trace should be regarded as reassuring.
- True early uniform decelerations are rare and benign, and therefore they are insignificant.
- Most decelerations in labor are variable.
- If a bradycardia occurs in the baby for more than 3 minutes, urgent medical aid should be sought and preparations should be made to urgently expedite the birth of the baby, classified as a category 1 birth. This could include moving the woman to theatre if the fetal heart has not recovered by 9 minutes. If the fetal heart recovers within 9 minutes, the decision to deliver should be reconsidered in conjunction with the woman if reasonable.
- A tachycardia in the baby of 160–180 bpm, where accelerations are present and no other adverse features appear, should not be regarded as suspicious. However, an increase in the baseline heart rate, even within the normal range, with other nonreassuring or abnormal features should increase concern.

As per the FIGO consensus guidelines on Intrapartum fetal monitoring: Cardiotocography, the following classification scheme may be used for interpretation and decision making in labor.

Parameter	***Normal***	***Suspicious***	***Pathological***
Baseline heart rate	110–160/min	Not within normal limits, but not pathological	<100/min
Variability	5–25/min	Not within normal limits, but not pathological	Reduced or increased variability or sinusoidal pattern
Deceleration	Not repetitive	Not within normal limits, but not pathological	• Repetitive late or prolonged decelerations • Over more than 30 min • Over 20 minutes with

Contd...

Contd...

Parameter	*Normal*	*Suspicious*	*Pathological*
			• One prolonged deceleration more than 5 minutes
Interpretation	No fetal hypoxia or acidosis	Low probability of fetal hypoxia or acidosis	High probability of fetal hypoxia or acidosis
Clinical management	No intervention needed to improve fetal oxygenation	Action required to correct reversible causes, close monitoring, more steps to rule out fetal hypoxia or acidosis	• Immediate action required to correct reversible causes. Expedite delivery if correction not possible • Immediate delivery in emergency situations like cord prolapse, placental abruption, uterine rupture

Note:
*There is uncertain significance attributed to absence of accelerations in labor
#Repetitive decelerations denote decelerations associated with >50% of uterine contractions

Q5. What are the indications for antepartum fetal surveillance? At what gestation should antepartum fetal surveillance be initiated? What is the recommended frequency of testing? Is there evidence that antepartum fetal surveillance decreases the risk of fetal demise or otherwise improves perinatal outcomes?

Draft recommendations:

- Antepartum fetal testing should be initiated at 32 0/7 weeks of gestation or later for most at-risk patients. In pregnancies with multiple or particularly worrisome high-risk conditions (e.g., chronic hypertension with suspected fetal growth restriction), testing might begin at a gestational age when delivery would be considered for perinatal benefit.
- There are no large clinical trials to recommend the frequency of antepartum fetal surveillance. If the maternal medical condition is stable and test results are reassuring weekly surveillance may be suggested in high-risk pregnancies. Surveillance can be increased in case of deteriorating maternal or fetal conditions or individualized in cases of multiple comorbidities.
- There should be shared decision making between the pregnant woman and her clinician regarding the timing and frequency of antepartum fetal monitoring in individuals at increased risk for still birth or with comorbidities.

- There is a paucity of evidence for the efficacy of antepartum fetal surveillance in low-risk women.
- Antenatal CTG should ideally be interpreted along with the a priori risk of fetal acidosis, Doppler ultrasonography, and biophysical profile and not as a standalone test for fetal well-being.

Evidence: American college of Obstetrics and Gynecology has come up with a ACOG committee opinion on Indications for outpatient antepartum fetal surveillance and they suggest that surveillance is needed for pregnant patient at increased risk of still birth of more than 0.8/1,000 pregnancies and are associated with an odds ratio for stillbirth of 2.0 compared with pregnancies without risk factors. However, they suggest that these are only guidance and not mandate and individualization about if and when to offer antenatal fetal surveillance is advised.

It is less likely that antenatal conventional cardiotocography may be beneficial in pregnancies at a low-risk of fetal acidosis.

Gaps in evidence: Cochrane systematic reviews of randomized controlled trials (RCTs) done by Grivell RM, in 2015 of the effectiveness of antenatal conventional CTG in preventing stillbirth, perinatal mortality, fetal loss and fetal death in women at increased risk suggest no clear benefit for mothers or their babies with regards to perinatal mortality, potentially preventable deaths, cesarean rates, Apgar scores less than seven at five minutes or admission to neonatal intensive care units. However, this evidence has low certainty as the trials were not of high quality, and were undertaken in the 1980s and 1990s. More studies are needed to see if outcomes for babies at increased risk of complications can be improved with antenatal CTG.

However, computerized CTG, on the other hand, shows a moderate certainty in reduction of risk of perinatal mortality in high-risk pregnancies.

Q6. Is the nomenclature for antenatal surveillance different from intrapartum surveillance?

Draft recommendations:

- The antenatal cardiotocography is also called as "non-stress test (NST)" and is performed in pregnancies that are at high risk of developing fetal hypoxia.
- The antenatal cardiotocography is not categorized and interpreted like intrapartum CTG and is reported as reassuring (reactive) versus nonreassuring NST (non-reactive). Any deviation from a reactive NST is defined as a non-reactive NST.

Evidence: The difference in the antenatal and intrapartum cardiotocography lies in the documentation of accelerations in the fetal heart rate of greater than 15 beats per minute for more than 15 seconds in response to fetal movements. It is performed over 20 minutes, but can be extended to 40 minutes to account for fetal sleep cycles.

Parameter	*Reactive*	*Nonreactive*
Baseline heart rate	110–160/min	Any deviation from reactive NST
Variability	5–25/min	
Accelerations	15 beats for 15 seconds 2 over a 20-minute period	Lack of sufficient accelerations over 40 minutes
Decelerations	None	May be present

Q7. CTG versus computerized CTG?

Draft recommendations: The computerized analysis of FHR is a promising solution for the reduction of adverse perinatal outcomes and elimination of inter- and intraobserver variability.

Evidence: The parameters of conventional cardiotocographic assessment apply for term fetuses. Preterm fetuses are likely to have false positive non-reactive NSTs to the tune of up to 50% at 24 weeks, to 15–20% at 28 to 32 weeks. The accelerations also have a lower amplitude of up to 10 beats per minute. The intra- and interobserver variation in interpretation of the conventional cardiotocography has been well documented. The computerized CTG helps to reduce observer variability. In addition, the objective determination of short-term variability (STV) and decelerations helps in the management of pregnancies with early onset fetal growth restriction (FGR).

Reduced STV is defined as variability less than 3.5 milliseconds before 29 weeks and less than 4 milliseconds thereafter.

Comparison of computerized CTG versus traditional CTG in the Cochrane systematic reviews of randomized controlled trials (RCTs) showed a significant reduction in perinatal mortality with computerized CTG.

Gaps: Tsipoura in his recent Systematic Review on Conventional Cardiotocography versus Computerized CTG Analysis and Perinatal Outcomes (2023) has not demonstrated a conclusive improvement in perinatal outcomes, no significant reduction in the rate of metabolic acidosis or obstetric interventions, with computerized CTG over conventional CTG; however, the elimination of observer variability gives a more reliable assessment with computerized CTG.

Further large-scale RCTs comparing cardiotocography with or without computerized analysis could be useful for the development of optimal strategies in daily clinical practice.

Q8. Is admission CTG useful in low-risk pregnancies?

Draft recommendations:

- The admission cardiotocograph (CTG) is a commonly used screening test consisting of a short (usually 20 minutes) recording of the fetal heart rate (FHR) and uterine activity performed on the mother's admission to the labor ward.
- Admission CTG should not be used for women who are low risk on admission in labor.
- Women should be informed that admission CTG is likely associated with an increase in the incidence of cesarean section without evidence of benefit.

Evidence: Contrary to continued use in clinical areas, Cochrane Database of Systematic Reviews of Cardiotocography versus intermittent auscultation of fetal heart on admission to labor ward for assessment of fetal wellbeing conducted by Devane D et al. suggests that admission CTG has not been found to improve outcomes in low-risk pregnancies as compared to intermittent auscultation. It has been associated with an increase in the cesarean section rate to the tune of 20%. There is no adequately powered data to conclusively detect differences in perinatal mortality between admission CTG and intermittent auscultation.

Q9. What medication will alter the FHR tracing for interpretation?

Draft recommendations: Fetal heart rate patterns can be influenced by the medications administered in the intrapartum period. Most often, these changes are transient, although they sometimes lead to obstetric interventions.

Medications that can affect the fetal heart rate are: Maternal administration of magnesium sulfate, CNS depressants like narcotics, barbiturates, and non-selective beta-blockers like propranolol have the potential to reduce heart rate reactivity on NST.

Epidural analgesia with local anesthetic agents (i.e., lidocaine, bupivacaine) can lead to sympathetic blockade, maternal hypotension, transient uteroplacental insufficiency, and alterations in the FHR.

Use of magnesium sulfate shows small changes in baseline, significant decrease in short-term variability but no decelerations. Caution should be used in ascribing unfavorable findings on EFM to the use of magnesium only.

The use of betamethasone transiently decreased the FHR variability, which returned to pretreatment status by the fourth to seventh day. There also may be a decrease in the rate of accelerations with the use of betamethasone.

Narcotics (75 mg meperidine, 10 mg morphine, 0.1 mg fentanyl, 10 mg nalbuphine) use decreases variability and causes a decrease in the frequency of accelerations.

Terbutaline: Increase in baseline FHR and incidence of fetal tachycardia.

Zidovudine: No difference in the FHR baseline, variability, number of accelerations.

Maternal smoking also shows a reduction in the fetal heart rate accelerations.

Physiological conditions like fetal sleep also may show no accelerations over a period of as long as 80 minutes.

Q10. Are intrauterine resuscitation measures useful for abnormal fetal heart tracing?

Draft recommendations:

- Intrauterine resuscitation measures have been shown to improve Category 2 and 3 CTG.
- Depending on the suspected underlying cause(s) of FHR abnormality, combining multiple interventions simultaneously may be appropriate and potentially more effective than doing individually or serially.

  A Category II or Category III FHR tracing requires evaluation of the possible causes and the methods of intrauterine resuscitation of proven benefit include the following:

  - Cervical examination to determine umbilical cord prolapse, rapid cervical dilation, or descent of the fetal head, fresh vaginal bleeding.
  - Monitoring maternal blood pressure level for evidence of hypotension, especially in those with regional anesthesia (if present, treatment with volume expansion or with ephedrine or both, or phenylephrine may be warranted).
  - Assessment of patient for uterine tachysystole by evaluating uterine contraction frequency and duration. Discontinue any labor stimulating agent like oxytocin if in use. In cases, not secondary to oxytocin infusion, the use of tocolytic agents may be considered to stop uterine contractions and perhaps avoid umbilical cord compression. A suggested regimen is subcutaneous terbutaline 0.25 mg.
  - Maternal repositioning into lateral or left or right lateral semi-recumbent position, reducing compression of the vena cava and improving uteroplacental blood flow. Avoid being supine.

Interventions of no or uncertain benefits:

- Do not offer intravenous fluids to treat fetal heart abnormalities unless the woman is hypotensive or has sign of sepsis.
- Prolonged use of maternal facial oxygen therapy may be harmful to the baby and should be avoided. There is no research evidence evaluating the benefits or risks associated with the short-term use of maternal facial oxygen therapy in cases of suspected fetal compromise.

- When the FHR tracing includes recurrent variable decelerations, amnioinfusion to relieve umbilical cord compression may be considered.

It is important to evaluate for the underlying cause(s) of the fetal heart rate pattern, as urgent delivery is necessary in some acute settings, such as uterine rupture, cord prolapse, or severe abruption. Physician judgment plays an important role in terms of assessing the probable cause, choosing the appropriate interventions for the specific patient setting, assessing the response to those interventions, and timing of cesarean delivery if the pattern persists.

Evidence: As per the ACOG practice bulletin on management of intrapartum fetal heart rate tracing, resuscitative interventions will depend on the type of FHR abnormalities.

For recurrent late decelerations, prolonged decelerations or bradycardia or minimal or absent fetal heart rate variability where fetal oxygenation and uteroplacental blood flow needs to improve, potential interventions include lateral positioning (either left or right), administer maternal oxygen and intravenous fluid bolus and reduce uterine contraction frequency has been suggested by ACOG. However, the NICE guidelines warn against maternal facial oxygen therapy as part of conservative measures because it may harm the baby. However, it can be used if it is given for maternal issues such as hypoxia, or as part of preoxygenation before a potential anesthetic.

Both ACOG and the NICE guidelines suggest that for tachysystole with Category 2 or 3 tracing, reducing uterine activity by discontinuing oxytocin or cervical ripening agents and need for tocolytic medication.

ACOG committee opinion on recurrent variable decelerations or prolonged decelerations or bradycardia, umbilical cord compression needs to be alleviated by initiating maternal repositioning or amnioinfusion. If prolapsed umbilical cord is noted, elevate the presenting fetal part while preparations are underway for operative delivery. The NICE on the other hand warns against the use of amnioinfusion.

NICE guidelines in 2022 also suggest not to offer intravenous fluids to treat fetal heart rate abnormalities unless the woman is hypotensive or has signs of sepsis. In case the woman is hypotensive secondary to an epidural top-up, start intravenous fluids, move her to a left lateral position, and call an anesthetist to review.

Q11. Are adjuncts to the use of continuous EFM including fetal scalp sampling useful in clinical practice?

Draft recommendations:

Adjuncts to the use of continuous EFM: Ancillary tests available that help to ensure fetal well-being in the face of a Category II or Category III FHR tracing, thereby reducing the high false-positive rate of EFM include:

- Fetal scalp sampling (fetal blood sampling)
- Allis clamp scalp stimulation

- Vibroacoustic stimulation
- Digital fetal scalp stimulation

Because vibroacoustic stimulation and digital scalp stimulation are less invasive than the other two methods, they are the preferred methods. When there is an acceleration following digital scalp stimulation and a sustained improvement in the CTG trace, acidemia is unlikely and labor can continue.

Where there is clear evidence of acute fetal compromise (for example, prolonged deceleration greater than 3 minutes), FBS should not be undertaken and urgent preparations to expedite birth should be made.

When a Category III FHR tracing is persistent, a scalp blood sample for the determination of pH or lactate may be considered. However, there is currently uncertainty around the usefulness of fetal blood sampling in predicting the outcomes for the baby and the mother during labor, and a wide variation in practice regarding its use.

The classification of fetal blood sample (FBS) results (NICE guidelines):

FBS result (pH)	***Interpretation***	***Response***
≥7.25	Normal FBS result	Repeat in 1 hour if FHR trace remains pathological
7.21–7.24	Borderline FBS result	Repeat in 1/2 hour if FHR trace remains pathological
≤7.20	Abnormal FBS result	Deliver

Contraindications to FBS include:

- Maternal infection (for example, HIV, hepatitis viruses and herpes simplex virus)
- Fetal bleeding disorders (for example, hemophilia)
- Prematurity (less than 34 weeks)

Evidence: Fetal blood sampling is a method of taking a blood sample from the fetal scalp, and is currently used in combination with cardiotocography during labor to assess the wellbeing of the fetus. Fetal blood sampling provides information on the pH and lactate levels of the fetal blood at the time of sampling, which in turn can be used to assess if the baby is receiving enough oxygen. This information can guide clinicians' decision-making regarding the appropriate steps for the ongoing management of labor, including the need to expedite birth. However, the process of fetal blood sampling is unpleasant for the woman and requires a skin prick on the baby's head.

Fetal scalp pH and scalp lactate may be measured through a scalp incision or by continuous scalp monitoring electrodes. However, this requires the cervix to be dilated to at least 3 cm and amniotomy followed by visualization of the scalp using an amnioscope for the collection of sample or placement of electrodes. The use of scalp pH assessment has decreased in clinical practice. The drawbacks of this technique include:

- Difficulty in obtaining and processing an adequate sample in a short period of time
- Contamination of sample by amniotic fluid or air
- Fetal infections and hemorrhage
- High cost of equipment
- Dislodgement of electrodes
- Expertise required
- Need for serial determinations
- Need for routine maintenance and calibration of laboratory equipment

More importantly, scalp stimulation, which is less invasive, provides similar information about the likelihood of fetal acidemia as does scalp pH. The sensitivity and positive predictive value of a low scalp pH to identify a newborn with hypoxic-ischemic encephalopathy was 50% and 3%, respectively. However, the greater utility of scalp pH is in its high negative predictive value (97–99%).

Fetal electrocardiography and ST-waveform analysis were developed in Sweden after extensive research. This too requires a scalp electrode placement. In addition, it shows no demonstrable difference in severe neonatal morbidity, mortality, and operative delivery rates as compared to CTG alone.

NICE during their review of literature compared fetal blood sampling plus CTG with CTG alone. They found no significant difference in neonatal outcomes namely neonatal encephalopathy, neonatal admission, or neonatal birth trauma. There was also no evidence of an important difference for modes of birth between the two groups. However, fetal blood sampling plus CTG had an important harm in terms of Apgar score less than 7 at 5 minutes.

Fetal blood sampling plus CTG was compared to digital fetal scalp stimulation plus CTG. The evidence for neonatal outcomes showed no important difference. There was also no evidence of any significant difference for instrumental vaginal births. When compared to digital fetal scalp sampling with CTG, fetal blood sampling with CTG showed an increase in cesarean births.

The NICE in its 2022 amendment suggests that if the CTG trace is suspicious with antenatal or intrapartum risk factors for fetal compromise, then consider digital fetal scalp stimulation. If this leads to an acceleration in fetal heart rate and a sustained improvement in the CTG trace, continue to monitor the fetal heart rate and clinical picture. Be aware that the absence of an acceleration in response to fetal scalp stimulation is a worrying sign that fetal compromise may be present, and that expedited birth may be necessary.

NICE is unable to make a recommendation about fetal blood sampling because of limited evidence.

Future developments: There is scope for more research in this topic as most of the studies included in the reviews and meta-analyses on cardiotocography have been performed in the decades between 1970 and 1990. In addition, the incidence of neonatal hypoxia, neonatal seizures, and cerebral palsy can be attributed to in utero antepartum insults that cannot be differentiated from the truly intrapartum causes due to their multifactorial nature. This reduces the prevalence of intrapartum causes of the above complications further, thus increasing the false positive rate and reducing the predictive value. On the other hand, electronic fetal monitoring is convenient, reducing the need for manpower, and the data can be stored electronically for decades, thus providing a safeguard from possible litigations. More high-powered studies in antepartum and intrapartum fetal surveillance along with improved sensitivity of equipment and reduced subjectivity or observer variability may improve the quality of data for extensive reviews and meta-analyses in the future.

CONCLUSION

Electronic fetal monitoring should be used as a tool to provide guidance on the fetal condition and must be interpreted together with the overall clinical picture including antenatal and existing or new intrapartum risk factors, maternal conditions, contraction frequency and the progress of labor and not as a standalone diagnostic test.

BIBLIOGRAPHY

1. Al Wattar BH, Honess E, Bunnewell S, et al. Effectiveness of intrapartum fetal surveillance to improve maternal and neonatal outcomes: a systematic review and network meta-analysis. CMAJ. 2021;193:E468.
2. Alfirevic Z, Devane D, Gyte GM, et al. Continuous cardiotocography (CTG) as a form of electronic fetal monitoring (EFM) for fetal assessment during labour. Cochrane Database Syst Rev. 2017;(2):CD006066.
3. American College of Obstetricians and Gynecologists. ACOG committee opinion: Indications for Outpatient antepartum fetal surveillance. Obstet Gynecol. 2021;137(6):e177-95.
4. American College of Obstetricians and Gynecologists. ACOG Practice Bulletin No. 106: Intrapartum fetal heart rate monitoring: nomenclature, interpretation, and general management principles. Obstet Gynecol. 2009;114(1):192-202.
5. American College of Obstetricians and Gynecologists. ACOG Practice Bulletin No. 116: Management of Intrapartum fetal heart rate tracings. Obstet Gynecol. 2010;116(5):1232-40.
6. Ayres-de-Campos D, Spong CY, Chandraharan E; FIGO Intrapartum Fetal Monitoring Expert Consensus Panel. FIGO consensus guidelines on intrapartum fetal monitoring: Cardiotocography. Int J Gynaecol Obstet. 2015;131(1):13-24.
7. Blix E, Brurberg KG, Reierth E, et al. ST waveform analysis vs. cardiotocography alone for intrapartum fetal monitoring: An updated systematic review

and meta-analysis of randomized trials. Acta Obstet Gynecol Scand. 2024;103(3):437-48.

8. Bohiltea RE, Mihai BM, Ducu I, et al. Current Innovative Methods of Fetal pH Monitoring-A Brief Review. Diagnostics (Basel). 2022;12(11):2675.
9. Devane D, Lalor JG, Daly S, et al. Cardiotocography versus intermittent auscultation of fetal heart on admission to labour ward for assessment of fetal wellbeing. Cochrane Database Syst Rev. 2017;1(1):CD005122.
10. Grivell RM, Alfirevic Z, Gyte GML, et al. Antenatal cardiotocography for fetal assessment. Cochrane Database Syst Rev. 2015;(9):CD007863.
11. Macones GA, Hankins GD, Spong CY, et al. The 2008 National Institute of Child Health and Human Development workshop report on electronic fetal monitoring: update on definitions, interpretation, and research guidelines. Obstet Gynecol. 2008;112:661-6.
12. NICE. National Institute for Health and Clinical Excellence guideline: Fetal monitoring in labour NG 229. [online] Available from www.nice.org.uk/guidance/ng229. [Last accessed November, 2024]
13. Rosen KG. Fetal electrocardiogram waveform analysis in labour. Curr Opin Obstet Gynecol. 2005;17:147-50.
14. Tsipoura A, Giaxi P, Sarantaki A, et al. Conventional Cardiotocography versus Computerized CTG Analysis and Perinatal Outcomes: a Systematic Review. Maedica (Bucur). 2023;18(3):483-9.
15. Umana OD, Siccardi MA. Prenatal Nonstress Test. In: StatPearls. Treasure Island (FL): StatPearls Publishing; 2023.
16. Vintzileos AM, Nochimson DJ, Guzman ER, et al. Intrapartum electronic fetal heart rate monitoring versus intermittent auscultation: a meta-analysis. Obstet Gynecol. 1995;85:149.